AN ESSAY ON
BINOCULAR VISION

AN ESSAY ON
BINOCULAR VISION

By

LORD CHARNWOOD

HAFNER PUBLISHING COMPANY
New York London
1965

Originally published 1950, London
Reprinted by Arrangement 1964

Printed and Published by
Hafner Publishing Company, Inc.
31 East 10th Street
New York, N.Y. 10003

Library of Congress Card Catalogue Number: 64-66329

Lithographed in the U.S.A.
by Noble Offset Printers, Inc.
New York, N. Y. 10003

CONTENTS

AUTHOR'S PREFACE

This little book is a monograph, in the true sense of the word, since it is written to record the views formed by one man as the outcome of his reading and his own experimental work. I started to write it solely as a thesis for the new higher diploma of the Worshipful Company of Spectacle Makers and as nearly half was written before I decided to offer it to a wider public and it was nearly finished before I decided to convert it from the first person, in which it was originally written, to the third person, many faults of style are in some measure due to this conversion.

A greater cause of untidiness of construction is the fact that I was still experimenting, reading, and changing my opinions up to the last moment and many results have had to be incorporated into chapters which I had thought finished until I read some newly published paper or designed some new experiment. I hope that these faults may be forgiven in a book which is not expected to have a permanent place in the literature, but is written in the hope that it may help other workers to go further. If someone else adds to our knowledge of the subject as a result of demolishing my views the trouble of putting them on paper will have been worthwhile.

One notable omission may call for some apology. There is no chapter on the psychology of binocular vision. The reason for this is that while I agree substantially with the views of the Gestalt school, I feel that they have lost their *raison d'être*. Though I feel that they had more of the truth than any other school, I have never been able to see that they had got any further than Tschermak and it seems to me that there is nothing in their theory which is not covered by Luneburg's *Mathematical Analysis of Binocular Vision*. Ames and his co-workers in the United States are opening up fresh fields in the psychology of vision which seem to me more likely to prove profitable but it is too early for me to attempt to comment. One fascinating question that I have only touched on in the text is: "What is the stimulus to accommodation?" It seems likely that this new work will throw much light on it.

Most sources of information are acknowledged in the text and the list of references. I wish to thank the Principal and Mr. C. L. Redding of the Northampton Polytechnic and my colleagues at the London Refraction Hospital for the facilities that they have given me. I also want to record my thanks to all the kind friends who have acted as guinea pigs in my experiments, particularly those who volunteered to submit to the annoyances inseparable from a prolonged occlusion test. Finally I want to record my indebtedness to Miss W. Georguli, of my own laboratory, not only for her ready participation in every experiment that we did and in coordinating the resulting data, but also for having undertaken all the routine work attendant on getting this book written.

CHARNWOOD.

September, 1950.

CHAPTER I

THE ANATOMICAL BASIS OF BINOCULAR VISION

In view of the specialised nature of this monograph, no attempt is made at a complete description of the eye as everyone who reads this will be fully familiar with its anatomy. This chapter will, therefore, deal only with those points which seem particularly relevant to the problems of binocular vision, with a minimum of context for the sake of continuity.

In considering binocular vision it seems logical to start with the two images on the retinæ. As the eyes are separated in space it is as well to notice at once that these two images can never be identical unless the eyes are looking at a scene so distant that it contains no element that is not sufficiently remote to make their separation negligible. The mechanism whereby the light falling on the receptors of the retina sets up nerve impulses is not relevant to our subject; it is, however, important to note that while there are about 7 million cones and about 125 million rods, there are only about one million ganglion cells with their axons which are the fibres of the optic nerves. Many observers put the number much lower.

In passing we should note that the ganglion cells are multipolar cells similar to those of the central nervous system, that their axons are finer than an ordinary peripheral nerve fibre, and that, though they have a medullary sheath after they have passed the lamina cribrosa, they resemble other fibres of the central nervous system in having no neurolemma. These facts serve to remind us that although it is convenient to regard it as the second cranial nerve, the optic nerve is not a true nerve but a fibre tract joining two portions of the central nervous system, and that the ganglion cells of the retina are neurones of the second order corresponding to cells in the nucleus gracilis or cuneatus.

It appears that at the centre of the fovea most, if not all, cones are in connection with a ganglion cell exclusive to themselves, yet the relative numbers of retinal receptors and optic nerve fibres make it clear that this is far from being the general rule, in the retina as a whole. Since the mind can have no means of knowing which receptor stimulated a given nerve fibre, when it connects with many, it is clear that the visual acuity of different parts of the retina must be a function of the number of nerve fibres leading from each part. Direct counting of the ganglion cell distribution is complicated by the fact that at the fovea there is considerable displacement of the ganglion cells, presumably for optical reasons. The generally accepted view is that the function of this thinning is to avoid the scattering of light as it passes through the inner layers of the retina. Walls (141) considers, from a study of avian foveæ, that it serves to enlarge the central image and that the human fovea is either immature or, more probably, degenerate. This theory is attractive as it helps to explain the extremely high visual acuity which some birds, such as kites and vultures, undoubtedly possess.

It is tempting to regard the ganglion cell layer and the layer of bipolar cells as two ganglions, analogous to ganglions in peripheral sensory nerves, but spread out in close relationship with the sensory endings. Unfortunately it is overwhelmingly probable that this view is far too simple, the neural structure of the retina is too elaborate and the variety of cells that make up these layers is too great, moreover not only are there cells whose sole function appears to be to effect cross connections between the bipolars and also between the ganglion cells, but there are also centrifugal fibres in the optic nerve bringing impulses back to the retina from higher centres. As we shall see later, these may subserve retinal inhibition.

Since there are at least three and almost certainly four or more distinct varieties of bipolar cell, Le Gros Clark has suggested that the different types of bipolar may serve to identify the three varieties of cone required by the three colour theory; while Polyak (113) believes that the cones are all of the same type responding to the whole of the visible spectrum and that the bipolars serve to analyse this general response into its three colour components by the different methods of their synaptic connections, these three components being synthesised again or integrated by the midget ganglion cells.

It is only necessary for our present purposes to consider these theories in so far as they bear on the resolving power of the eye. Both of them seem to require that the acuity of vision should be substantially less for monochromatic light than for white light which, as Hartridge and others have shown, is not the case; moreover, the structure of the foveal area of the retina where colour perception and visual acuity are at their highest does not seem to accord well with either theory. At the fovea an enormous number of cones appear to employ a pure or private cone path, one cone in synaptic relation with one midget bipolar cell, and this, in its turn, in relation with one midget ganglion cell, in addition one type of bipolar cell—the mop variety—if not altogether missing—must be extremely rare in the rod free area as it has never been observed there. It seems more probable that the midget bipolars which are typically in relation with one cone and one ganglion cell serve to transmit a colourless form sense which is responsible for the visual acuity of the eye to all colours, while the diffuse bipolars which make connection with several cones modify and colour the image. The fact that the only two varieties of bipolar available have not been shown to be distinct does not seem to be of great consequence as there is no reason why the cells serving different colour sensations should be morphologically different, nor are many varieties needed if we accept a theory akin to Hering's opponent colour theory. Granit's (66) work, in which he has shown that some fibres at least transmit on and off impulses, also seems to support this hypothesis, as does Hartridge's (67) observation of small groups of cones in the fovea which respond to colourless stimulus with a coloured sensation, and it is possible that the diffuse bipolars are the explanation of his cluster hypothesis.

It seems impossible to accept Polyak's contention that the midget bipolars are the integrators of colour sensation as this is, in effect, placing the " conscious " cell in the retina and requires that the optic nerve-fibres be capable of transmitting impulses which vary in quality as well as magnitude, which is at variance with all that is known of the transmission of nerve impulses. It seems likely that if the " conscious " cells for colour were located in the retina, a man who had bilateral optic atrophy or had lost both eyes would lose all conception of colour, which we know is not the case.

Very little is known of the functions of the centrifugal fibres, the centrifugal bipolars or the horizontal and amacrine association cells. It is possible that one of them may be responsible for the antichromatic responses. Unless they subserve inhibition the centrifugal bipolars seem the likeliest structures for this task as they appear to be common at the fovea, though they are also present at the periphery.

The fovea centralis, or rod-free area of the retina, has a diameter of about 0·5 mm. which subtends an angle of about 1° 40′ (113). Various authorities have given slightly different values but they all agree fairly closely. In this area there are some thirty thousand cones, with a probable centre to centre distance of about 3μ. Polyak puts the diameter of the foveal cones as low as 1—1·5μ, while Kölliker puts it as high as 5μ. Hartridge accepts 3μ as the most probable separation which corresponds to 2 mm. at ten metres, or 41 seconds of arc, which he calls a cone unit.

The optic nerves decussate at the chiasma so that fibres from the right hand part of the visual field of each eye pass to the left optic tract and vice versa, but there is no splitting of fibres, nor are the impulses from the two eyes brought together there. The optic tracts pass on and spread over the lateral geniculate bodies and it seems certain that all the true visual fibres relay here. Something under 10 per cent pass on and form a cell station under the lateral margin of the superior colliculus, the pretectal nucleus. The new relay fibres from these cross partly in the posterior commissure ventral to the iter, while some pass direct and uncrossed to the sphincter centre in the anterior part of the third nerve nucleus, probably in the accessory nucleus of Edinger-Westphal, and so relay on to the ciliary ganglion.

The lateral geniculate bodies of primates show a well defined six layer structure. Minchowski (103) was the first to report in 1920 that section of one optic nerve caused degeneration in alternate layers in the monkey. This was confirmed by Le Gros Clark who showed that the crossed fibres end in laminæ 1, 4 and 6, while the uncrossed end in laminæ 2, 3 and 5. He further showed that this was also true in the human brain. Le Gros Clark and Penman (90) showed that there is at least an approximate point-to-point projection of the retina. Polyak (113a) has shown the minimal cortical lesion leads to degeneration in all six layers, while a minimal retinal lesion always affects the appropriate three layers. Glees and Le Gros Clark (88) showed that each fibre of the optic tract ended in a spray, or five or six terminal buttons, each button being in relation to one cell of the lateral geniculate body and only one button was ever found in relation with any cell in the small celled laminæ unlike the lower animals such as the cat, where Glees (65) has found 30 to 40 such buttons to one geniculate cell. In this respect, the cells of the primate lateral geniculate stand in strong contrast to cells of the spinal cord, medulla and cerebellum. Layers 1 and 2 have cells substantially larger than the other four and since the 5 or 6 spray termination has not been demonstrated in them it must be considered unlikely.

Le Gros Clark (85) has also shown that the laminar structure of the lateral geniculates cannot be imposed on them by the geography of the optic tracts as the crossed and uncrossed fibres seem to be arranged quite at random there, and no segregation appears to take place until the tracts reach the geniculates where fibres may be seen passing straight through several layers before reaching their final destination. These investigations led to the conclusion that there are about 1,600,000 cells in the small celled laminæ, and 200,000 in the large celled laminæ of the Macaque monkey. On the assumption that each fibre of the optic tract ends in relation with the 5 or 6 cells in the small celled laminæ, it seems that they represent the destination of about 290,000 retinal fibres, while the large celled laminæ cannot be the destination of more than 200,000.

Balado and Franke (8) (quoted by Clark) claim that the number of cells in the human geniculate is very much less, 480,000 in the small celled laminæ, and 86,000 in the large, and that each cell corresponds to a retinal fibre. The actual number of retinal fibres shows great variation between individuals. Bruesch and Arey have recorded numbers ranging roughly from half a million to well over a million, though it must be remembered that these figures include the light reflex fibres and the centrifugal ones. It is almost certain that the optic nerves of some monkeys contain more fibres than those of man, and, indeed, in some species the visual apparatus as a whole appears to be more highly refined.

Despite the fact that many authors have described descending fibres from the occipital cortex to the geniculate, the evidence against them seems to be overwhelming. Complete ablation of one lobe of the occipital cortex in the monkey causes all cells of the lateral geniculate to degenerate. Only one type of cell has been demonstrated in each lamina and the rapidity with which degeneration of these cells follows, on section of the optic nerve, strongly suggests that in the higher species they have no other source of stimulation to maintain their activity. The lateral geniculates therefore appear to be simply relay stations where some topographical rearrangement of fibres occurs but no fresh impulses are impressed to modify those arising from the retina.

From the fact that retinal lesions always lead to cell atrophy in three layers of the lateral geniculate, it would seem that the conducting unit is a three fibre one, while the degeneration in all six from the smallest cortical lesion suggests a six fibre conducting unit, though the absence of any intercalated neurons between the laminæ shows that the point-to-point representation of the separate uniocular images is preserved as far as the cortex, and that it is only at this level that they are brought into relation.

It has been suggested that the large cells of laminæ 1 and 2 may be connected with the large ganglion cells of the retina, and the small cells of the remaining layers with the midget ganglion cells. The chief ground for this suggestion being that they bear similar numerical relationships. The fact that the large celled laminæ are fully developed only in the higher primates and that the midget ganglion cells reach their full specialisation only in the same group tells against this hypothesis. Le Gros Clark has suggested that there may be a connection between the three fibre conducting unit of the optic nerve, as shown by the structure of the lateral geniculates and the trichromatic theory of colour vision. To test this he kept three monkeys in red light completely free from blue radiations for a month and then killed them and examined their lateral geniculates. In two cases he found marked degeneration of the macular region in lamina 1 only, i.e. only crossed fibres being affected. No change could be found in the remaining monkey. It is difficult to see how the blue-free light could affect crossed fibres only, or why it should be selective to the macula; the anatomy of the chiasma suggests that some local condition is the more probable explanation and the hypothesis must be regarded as unproved.

The retinal impulses relayed in the lateral geniculate body are carried back in the optic radiations which end in or near the white line of Gennari in the area striata of the occipital cortex. It is probable that all, or nearly all, of the optic radiations end in the granular layer which separates the outer layer of pyramidal cells from the deeper ganglion layer and the lamina multiformis which contains the solitary cells of Meynert.

It is certain that each fibre of the optic radiations ends in relation to a large number of granule cells, and that the granule cells stimulated by the two retinæ are intimately mingled, as the smallest lesion of the visual cortex leads to degeneration in all six layers of the lateral geniculate. It is here, therefore, that the two uniocular images are brought together for the first time and it is presumably this area striata that provides the physiological basis for the fusion of the two uniocular images and probably also for stereopsis. The evidence from clinical observation is that it is a purely perceptive area and that all retinal impulses must pass through it in order to reach consciousness.

Perception of colour, relative direction and discrimination of form are all functions of the striate area; the parastriate and the peristriate areas around it are assumed to be the visuo-psychic, or visual memory centres. Holmes has shown that agnosia of letters is produced by a lesion involving the lateral and inferior surface of the occipital lobe close to the striate area. For reasons which will be considered later, the writer thinks it extremely probable that the striate area performs the integrations necessary to frame one three-dimensional impression from the two uniocular images, and possibly the modification, or even rejection, of the result in order to make it conform to the dictates of experience and the evidence from conflicting uniocular clues.

It used to be taught that the visual cortex was directly connected with many other cortical areas, particularly those of the parietal lobe, by well defined systems of association fibres. Doubt was first aroused when Le Gros Clark and Northfield (89) excised almost the whole parietal cortex of a monkey. The animal was allowed to survive for two months, which would be ample time to show cytological changes in the visual cortex from the severing of association fibres, if such existed. However, no such changes could, in fact, be demonstrated, and the lamina pyramidalis, to which neuro-anatomists assign association fibres, showed its full normal cell population.

Le Gros Clark (85) decided to extend this research by studying, by Marchi degeneration methods, the results of operative lesions of the occipital cortex of monkeys. The two main classes of fibres found in the visual cortex are a diffuse plexus of oblique fibres largely derived from the optic radiations and the radial fibres running vertically in discrete bundles. In these experiments well marked tracts of efferent fibres were shown, which appeared to belong to two main systems leading down into the brain stem and are believed to be cortico pontine and cortico tectal. At the time Clark thought it possible that some might be cortico geniculate, but this later work makes this extremely improbable. No association fibres leading to the parietal lobes, or any other distant parts of the cortex, have been found, though evidence was found for association fibres running into the peristriate, cortex area 18. For the rest, no association fibres longer than 4 or 5 mm. were demonstrated. In some previous work Le Gros Clark and Sunderland (91) found that only about 15 per cent of the radial fibres had undergone degeneration when a strip of visual cortex 6 mm. wide had been isolated for over four months. Putting these two results together, it seems that the majority of fibres in each radial bundle originate in cortical cells not more than a very few millimetres away. It follows that in the first stages the activation of distant cortical areas from the visual cortex must be by relays of short neurons.

These results agree with those obtained by Dusser de Barenne and W. S. McCulloch (52) by local strychninization and recording electro-corticograms. Local strychninization of many frontal areas produces effects in various distant regions, but in the area striata they only recorded the characteristic strychnine spikes in the actual area strychninized and its immediate neighbourhood, regions more than 1 or 2 mm. away remaining quiet.

The solitary cells of Meynert in the lamina multiformis have already been mentioned. These are large cells having horizontal dendrites spreading over a relatively large area. It is more than likely that their axons are among the efferent fibres recorded by Le Gros Clark in his Marchi degeneration experiments, as he has since shown (86) that they undergo degeneration if the cortico mesencephalic fibres are cut. They probably mediate rapid mass reactions of the cortex and are at least partly responsible for involuntary movements towards fixation and for its maintenance. Cortico mesencephalic fibres form well defined fasciculi penetrating the base of the pulvinar and entering the deeper part of the stratum opticum of the superior colliculus; to what extent they originate in the striate area and to what extent in the peristriate is doubtful.

Stimulation of the frontal lobes produces eye movements, though the path of the fibres to the oculo-motor nuclei is unknown. Wolff (150) says that it probably runs with the pyramidal tract; complete decussation, probably in the posterior commissure, has been proved. Stimulation of the visual cortex also produces conjugate eye movements, but if the frontal motor centre is stimulated simultaneously in a position which causes movement in the opposite direction, the resulting movement will be that corresponding to this stimulation and not that which would be evoked by stimulation of the occipital cortex alone (105). It follows that somewhere fibres from both occipital and frontal lobes make synaptic relation with the same neuron in order that one may be able to inhibit the other, but whether this occurs in the oculo-motor nuclei, or at some higher level, is not clear. Gordon Holmes (75) says, " All evidence at our disposal indicates that the frontal oculo-motor centre is concerned in those movements and reactions of the eyes which we call voluntary. Through an effort of will we can turn our eyes in any direction and converge them on a near object . . . the functions of the occipital centre are more numerous. Fusion, that is the reactions necessary to unify the separate impressions from the two retinæ, and accommodation depend on it. The movement of the eyes to an object outside central vision, insofar as it is voluntary, is also excited through the occipital cortex by extra-foveal impulses. And finally, the maintenance of fixation on a point, whether it is at rest or in movement, is determined by a cortical reflex mechanism in the occipital lobes."

The oculo-motor nuclei lie in the midbrain in the floor, or ventral to the fourth ventricle at about the level of the colliculi. The third nerve nucleus, the topmost, consists of two paired columns of cells some 7 mm. in length, lying just dorsally to the posterior longitudinal bundles, joined by bridges of cells to a central unpaired group, chiefly of large motor cells, the nucleus of Perlia. In close association are two paired columns of small cells, the Edinger-Westphal nuclei. Another pair of groups of similar small cells, the nuclei of Darkschewitsch may be mentioned in passing. It is now generally assumed that they serve some non-ocular function (38). There is also some doubt whether the Edinger-Westphal nuclei have any ocular function; they do not contain typical motor cells, section of N III does not result in their retrograde degeneration and the destruction of the Edinger-Westphal nuclei has not resulted in loss of pupillary function (62).

Immediately below the nuclei of the third nerve, and almost part of it, is that of the fourth. Not only are they close together but their interconnection has been proved by the fact that electro stimulation of the caudal extremity of the third nerve nucleus has caused intorsion of the contralateral eye (15). The fourth nerve is unique among motor nerves in making a complete, or almost complete decussation to emerge on the dorsal side of the brain stem. Various theories have been advanced to account for this abnormality which is of great antiquity phylogenetically, as it is present throughout almost the whole of the animal kingdom. Ontogenetically, it is differentiated very early in embryonic life. Perhaps the most attractive theory is that it was originally the sensory nerve of the segment of which the third nerve was the motor nerve; some colour is given to this hypothesis by Gaskell's claim (150) that there are vestiges of a degenerated ganglion near its origin. Its nucleus consists chiefly of large motor cells of some 40—50μ diameter, but, as with the third, there are also some small cells.

The nuclei of the sixth nerve also lie in the floor of the fourth ventricle immediately laterally to the posterior lateral bundles. They are situated further caudally than the other oculo-motor nuclei in the immediate vicinity of the diffuse complex of cells which make up the eighth or vestibular nucleus. It is considered likely that the centre for conjugate lateral gaze may lie in this neighbourhood (38).

This seems to be the logical place for a brief digression in order to discuss what is meant by the words nucleus and centre. In a purely anatomical sense the word nucleus is quite unequivocal; it means a more or less defined mass of cells where the final synaptic connections of a nerve occur. In the case of a motor nerve, it is the location of the cells whose axons constitute the nerve fibres. In the case of a sensory nerve, the nerve fibres have their cell station in the ganglion and the nucleus is the cell station of the next neuron in the chain. In every case it is the start or end of a common path, motor or sensory. Only in the case of the cranial nerves can separate and distinct nuclei for the individual nerves be located, in the spinal nerves they are inextricably intermingled in the grey matter of the cord.

Sherrington (125) has shown that a complete reflex arc can operate at a nuclear or equivalent level, for example, the scratch reflex in the spinal dog, but we have also seen that even so well defined and highly differentiated a body of cells as the lateral geniculate may be nothing more than a relay station.

Confining our attention to motor nuclei, we can say with certainty that they represent the last link to the final common path. The reinforcement or inhibition of motor impulses may take place at this level but no later. It does not follow that any co-ordination does take place there. By analogy, a motor nerve nucleus may be nothing more than a junction box where several control mechanisms can send impulses down a multi-conductor cable with a safety interlock to ensure that only one control mechanism can take command at any one moment. This view is strongly suggested by Sherrington's investigations of the scratch reflex. In general the histological organisation of a nucleus is far too simple for it to seem likely that it is, in itself, a co-ordinating centre.

The nucleus of the third nerve is particularly interesting in that it is more highly organised than most and that the nerve innervates a number of interacting muscles. At one time it seemed safe to locate the control of each muscle in a definite portion of the nucleus. Bernheimer's scheme based on retrograde degeneration experiments on monkeys has long been the most generally accepted. According to this analysis the connections from front to rear are the levator, the superior rectus, the medial rectus, the inferior oblique, and the inferior rectus; the front portions innervating the homolateral eye, the middle both eyes and the rear portions, the contralateral. There is some clinical evidence for this arrangement and a little against it; however, clinical evidence from the postmortem examination of cases of long standing is never very satisfactory for such purposes. Bender and Weinstein (15) have re-examined the question with the Horsley-Clarke electrical stimulation technique and their provisional results suggest a very different arrangement. They found no evidence of any control of the contralateral eye from this nucleus, but downward movements of the eye resulting from stimulation of the dorsal-oral extremity and upward movements with retraction of the upper lid from stimulating the caudal ventral extremity. Danis (46) gets similar results on the cat.

It has been argued that there is no fixed location of function within the nucleus, and the fact that patients who have had slips from the superior and inferior recti transplanted to supplement or replace a paralysed lateral rectus, can abduct, has been adduced in support of this hypothesis. This assumption is certainly a convenient way of reconciling the conflicting results of Bernheimer and of Bender and Weinstein, but results from such transplants need very careful interpretation, and against it is the so-called pseudo-Graefe phenomenon where after section of the third nerve, if the stumps have not been properly aligned, nerve fibres which originally ran to the inferior rectus may regenerate into the levator causing a retraction of the upper lid when the patient attempts to look down. This phenomenon is permanent. It seems reasonable to assume that the location of the cells innervating each muscle is definite and immutable and to accept that it has not as yet been fully worked out.

The definition of a " centre " is far more difficult. Perhaps the best description would be that region of the brain where a movement is designed and from which the necessary impulses to originate the appropriate contraction of agonist and inhibition of antagonist muscles are transmitted to the appropriate motor nuclei. The existence of a function does not appear to prove the existence of a centre for performing it; for instance, there can be no question that the eyes can be diverged in the interests of fusion, and in certain rare cases for the avoidance of fusion, but no divergence centre has ever been demonstrated, nor does it seem necessary to postulate one. On the other hand, phylogenetic and ontogenetic evidence both strongly suggest that the central nucleus of Perlia is connected with convergence, as does some clinical evidence. The acceptance of this does not of necessity involve accepting it as a convergence centre, as we have defined one, though it is commonly accepted as such.

The cerebral cortex appears to be by far the most flexible part of the central nervous system, and the higher we go in the phylogenetic scale the greater that flexibility becomes. The astonishing recovery of function that can follow destructive lesions, or the operative removal of large areas of the cortex, has been held to show that, within limits, any portion of the cortex can perform the functions of any other provided that it has sufficiently direct access to the necessary final common path. This does not in the least deny the existence of centres for individual functions, but it does imply that their localisation from post mortem material can be very uncertain.

The work of Le Gros Clark, that we have quoted above, explains quite clearly why no recovery follows the loss of vision from lesions of the striate area and the agnosia and comparable defects following injury to the neighbouring cortex. Since there are no long association fibres from the area striata to other parts of the cortex and association is performed by relays of short neurons within the cortex itself, it follows that destruction of either the visual cortex or an association area cuts off the rest of the cortex from the necessary final common path.

The phrase " final common path " was originally used by Sherrington of motor paths and is still usually so used, but it seems reasonable, in the present context, to use it " in reverse " to describe an afferent pathway whose destruction blocks all access for the impulses, necessary for the continuance of some function, to the rest of the cortex.

We may assume that different functions are integrated in different portions of the brain. It seems that voluntary eye movements originate in the frontal cortex but are represented there as a movement of the eyes not as a contraction of one muscle and the inhibition of its antagonist.

This also seems to be true of other bodily movements. It even seems probable that ocular movements originating in the occipital cortex are represented there, as a change in the object of attention rather than as a movement. These impulses are analysed into their component muscle movements and the voluntary and involuntary movements are selected or integrated in centres in the brain stem. It has been suggested that some involuntary movements may have, in addition, private paths to the motor nuclei for use under imperative stimuli. This possibility appears less likely since Rademaker and Ter Braak (115) have shown that the blinking reflex in response to a threat, one of the fastest, is abolished by removal of the striate area, or the appropriate motor cortex.

As we have already noted, conjugate lateral deviations of the eyes result from stimulation of the contralateral frontal motor cortex. Stimulation of the upper portion of the area results in a downward component in the deviation and similarly an upward component results from stimulation of the lower portions. In order to cause a directly upwards or downwards movement it is necessary to stimulate the two cerebral hemispheres symmetrically so long as the centres for lateral gaze and their connections are intact (105).

It is abundantly clear that the centre for conjugate lateral gaze is in the pontine region and the weight of evidence seems to suggest that it may be that portion of the vestibular nucleus which is concerned with eye movements. The early stage of evolution at which vestibular impulses serve to maintain the direction of gaze steady during body movements lends colour to this hypothesis and Spiegel (127) has shown that the destruction of this nucleus abolishes lateral conjugate eye movements from stimulation of either the frontal or occipital cortex. It has been suggested that the sixth nerve nuclei are themselves the centre, but their cell content does not seem large enough to serve this function. Cogan quotes Garel 1882, and Hunnius 1881 as stating that the sixth nucleus can degenerate without leading to degeneration in the third nucleus. In view of the early date of these observations, this may be the result of inadequate technique since A. Rochon-Duvigneand (117) in " Les Yeux et la Vision des Vertebre " quotes J. Deverine as having demonstrated fibres myelinating very early (and therefore of great antiquity) as running in the posterior longitudinal bundle, springing from the small cell elements, and interconnecting the sixth nucleus to the homolateral third.

The location of the subcortical centre for vertical movements seems much more surely established. The only evidence for their representation in the basal ganglion, or reticular substance, is the fact that vertical paresis is common in Parkinson's disease and some other affections. Against this there is a great bulk of anatomical and experimental evidence to locate this function in the superior colliculi. Fibres have been traced to it both from the occipital cortex (73) and to the third and fourth nerve nuclei Costaldi (Costaldi, L., quoted by Cogan). Hoessly (73) has produced vertical eye movements by its electric stimulation, confirming a result reported by earlier workers. Its destruction abolishes, or greatly reduces, vertical movements from stimulation of the occipital cortex, though it appears to have little effect on those resulting from stimulation of the frontal cortex (128). It seems clear, however, that the superior colliculi are not the only centres concerned in vertical eye movements, both from the fact that we have just noted, that their destruction does not abolish the effects of stimulating the frontal lobes and that vestibular control can survive lesions that have destroyed voluntary and fixation control, as is seen in the "doll's head" movements sometimes seen under the influence of the otolith reflexes (59), when the paralysis of vertical movements is otherwise complete, as in Huntington's chorea. The fact that movements due to other stimuli are unimpaired disposes of any suggestion that effects attributed to the superior colliculi are in reality due to injury to, or accidental stimulation of, the third nerve nuclei. Since the nucleus is the start of the final common path, its injury or destruction must affect all movements of the muscle, however initiated, and retention of one function shows that part, at least, of the final common path is intact. Holmes (74) gives clinical grounds for agreeing with these locations for the centres of conjugate lateral and vertical gaze. He also denies the existence of any true motor centre in the occipital cortex, which he regards as a higher ocular reflex centre as well as a perceptive area. This seems to me to be very much the same as the suggestion made above. It is clear that the motor cells for eye movements are not located in any part of the cortex; movements in response to stimulation of the frontal cortex must be due to the stimulation having simulated the will to make that movement, while stimulation of the occipital cortex has simulated a visual stimulus.

There is some evidence to suggest that the colliculi may have pupillary connections, but as these have no direct bearing on stereopsis we will not discuss them, nor will we enter into details of pupillary innervation at any other stage.

The remaining conjugate movement is the rotation of the eyes, clockwise and counterclockwise, which tends to cancel out head tilts, a head tilt of 45° resulting in a wheel rotation of the eyes of about 37° in the opposite direction (Kompanejetz, quoted by Cogan). So far as is known, torsions have no representation in the frontal lobes but they may be represented in the occipital lobes as slight torsional following movements can be elicited by rotating the visual field, and cyclo-fusional movements are well known. According to Cogan, Javal was the first to have called attention to torsional movements which he noticed through finding that his cylindrical lenses no longer corrected his astigmatism when his head was tilted, while Duke-Elder claims the discovery for his fellow-countryman, John Hunter. Apart from fusional and following torsions, wheel rotations of the eyes are mediated exclusively by the labyrinths. Grahe has reported that destruction of one labyrinth chiefly affects the results of tilting the head to the opposite side, while Kompanejetz states that destruction of both labyrinths abolishes torsion of the eyes completely.

In addition to the conjugate eye movements that we have been considering, there are the disjugate movements that the eyes perform in the interests of fusion, convergence, divergence, and cyclovergence. Cogan suggests a distinction between convergence of equal innervation obeying Hering's Law and fusional movements which may be measured as ductions, on the grounds that these movements occur much more slowly than other eye movements, and that the induced position tends to persist. As we shall see, when we come to consider phorias, there is some doubt whether these fusional " movements " are purely eye movements, or whether they are partly a cortical readjustment. From both clinical observation and from subjective impressions, from experiment on himself, this distinction seems to the writer to be a real one. Whether these purely fusional movements are the result of equal innervations, as postulated by Hering, or whether they should be regarded as monocular is an open question. The writer's opinion is that the innervation is binocular on the grounds that a prism placed base-in before one eye seems to shift the position of the fixation point by approximately half the amount that two such prisms with their base-apex lines pointing in the same direction would; however, the observation is not quantitative and is certainly inconclusive. In his view, the best evidence for uniocular innervations for ductions is Bielchowsky's dissociated vertical divergence; however, since an upward movement of one eye and a downward movement of the other does not exist alone, as a normal function of human, frontally directed eyes, it is dangerous to argue from it to lateral movements.

The most important of the disjunctive movements is convergence; its investigation is more difficult than that of the conjugate movement because it is not nearly so well developed in any of the laboratory animals as it it is in man, with the result that even less is known about the centres and pathways involved than is known in the case of the conjugate movements. Numerous writers have reported convergence as resulting from stimulation of both the frontal and occipital cortex, but almost always from bilateral stimulation, and their observations seem such as to suggest that the convergence observed was the result of simulating a normal cortical stimulus rather than of stimulating a convergence centre directly (105), (120), (121).

While it is easy to initiate voluntary convergence by looking at an imaginary point, particularly one on the midline, most people find it impossible to do this if there is a real object near but not at the intended point of convergence. This clearly suggests that the occipital lobes dominate the frontal lobes for convergence. Normally convergence, accommodation, and pupil contraction occur together as one function. It is said that the pupil will contract in co-operation with either of the other two movements if one is prevented from acting normally. Since pupil contraction is a purely involuntary function innervated by the autonomic nervous system, association with the other two functions presumably occurs in the mid-brain. However, since convergence can be retained when all lateral movements are paralysed (116), it is reasonable to suppose that convergence impulses reach the oculo-motor nuclei at the level of the superior colliculi rather than via the pons. This supposition may be supported by the fact that convergence and depression are associated to some extent, as is shown by the change of near phoria that accompanies depression of the eyes. The fact that the superior colliculi appear to be the mid-brain centres for upward and downwards gaze, also tends to make this assumption seem plausible. This could be a purely mechanical effect resulting from the line of action of the inferior recti; however, the fact that raising the eyes above the primary position makes voluntary deviation easier and not more difficult makes this suggestion seem very unconvincing, since the line of action of the superior recti is symmetrical with that of the inferior.

Perlia's nucleus, the median unpaired group of motor cells which forms part of the third nerve nucleus complex, is generally assumed to be the final centre for convergence, chiefly on phylogenetic grounds. It is fully developed only in man, who has by far the most highly developed powers of convergence of any animal. In the lower mammals and vertebrates below the mammals, the two third nerve nuclei are quite separate, and as we ascend the scale the accessory nuclei of Edinger-Westphal appear as a median unpaired structure before the two main nuclei fuse. Such a central nucleus is well defined in the rabbit (21). In the seal, the bridge joining the main nuclei is well established, though the Edinger-Westphal nuclei are still only represented as a scattered, ill-defined colony of small cells, and they are still unpaired in the cat. Stutterheim has described the cat as having a central nucleus of Perlia and has said that the feline are the lowest mammals to possess the power of convergence, denying that dogs possess it. The writer thinks it likely that he mistook this unseparated Edinger-Westphal cell complex for the forward projection of the bridge between the third nuclei which is the true central nucleus. In addition, the statement that dogs have no powers of convergence is incorrect; the writer has repeatedly observed it in them.

It is generally considered that the accessory nuclei of Edinger-Westphal are concerned with pupil size variations and accommodation. Except for the assistance that it gives in attempts to elucidate the localisation of function in the brain, the former is of no interest for our immediate study, and it seems logical to leave the latter on one side until we have completed our discussion of the innervation of the extraocular muscles.

While the combined influences of depression and accommodation cause the two eyes to be directed approximately to the object of regard, experience with the Maddox wing and such instruments shows that this convergence is by no means exact. Moreover, most people show at least some small phoria when the eyes are dissociated, even when looking into the distance. It seems reasonable then to agree with Cogan in classing fusional movements as something apart from the rest of the eye movements. Bielchowsky (16) also classifies eye movements under the headings:—1. Voluntary. 2. Fusional. 3. Reflex. The only movements which he regards as purely reflex are those of vestibular and proprioceptive origin, saying that they alone are entirely subcortical. The same is, however, true of the elevation of the eyes with the closure of the lids. Convergence and its inhibition are, as we have seen, in some measure under voluntary control. He describes the fusional movements as psycho-optical reflexes, claiming that (*i*) they are independent of the will and take place only in response to adequate fusible stimuli; (*ii*) they can be developed and will increase, over a series of tests, to a limit which cannot be passed, though training may hasten reaching this limit; (*iii*) the power of fusion varies greatly from individual to individual, and for the same individual from one occasion to the next, depending on his physical and mental fitness and freshness; (*iv*) the innervation does not relax immediately after stimulation has ceased but fades gradually.

The writer's own subjective sensations of divergent fusional movements certainly bear out all that he says. While it is possible to assist the fusional movements both by relaxing one's accommodation and by assuming the most favourable head posture, there is no escaping conviction that, with a suitable image separation, when one has brought the images as far as one can, some force quite divorced from one's will takes over and achieves fusion. This does not conflict, in his view, with one's controlled and voluntary ability to break fusion on near objects by voluntary relaxation or by voluntary over convergence.

The writer's descriptions of subjective or introspective sensations on fusional movements are based on divergent fusional movements, as he happens to find divergence easier to initiate and control than convergence, and therefore finds such experiments more amenable to introspection, but it seems reasonable to assume that convergent, divergent, and cyclo-fusional movements are similar in all essentials. In considering these fusional movements it is important to bear in mind the complication, which we have already noticed, which retinal slip may introduce.

This leaves us with the vexed question of whether there is, or is not, a divergence centre in the brain. The most generally accepted theory is that divergence is brought about solely by the relaxing of convergence, primarily in conjunction with accommodation which may subsequently be exercised alone. The evidence for a distinct centre for divergence is far from adequate (22). It rests chiefly on a few reported clinical cases of paralysis of divergence as an isolated function (51), (14). In addition, the writer has reported a case (30) of a patient who steadily maintained a manifest 15° divergent strabismus despite the fact that her eyes were straight under cover, the divergence occurring only when both eyes were uncovered. Several other cases of disjunctive movements to avoid fusion have been reported, but this is the only case that he knows of where such an antifusional movement was one of divergence. (He has since seen another such case, but the divergence was only 5°.) We will return to the consideration of these antifusional movements later.

In the lower vertebrates and many of the lower mammals propriocep-tion from the muscles of the neck and trunk muscles plays an important part in the movement of the eyes. In man, with his highly developed voluntary eye movements, these reflexes have become so overlaid with later ones and other functions as to have become virtually extinguished. They can be demonstrated fairly easily in a premature baby and with rather more difficulty in a full term infant. There are a few cases reported in the literature of their having been demonstrated in adult pathological cases where other reflexes were lost. It is quite clear that they cannot have any important bearing on the latest and most refined form of vision, so a discussion of them would be out of place in this monograph.

The labyrinthine influences on the eye movements in man are of greater importance, though they also, for the most part, are sufficiently subordinated to the overriding influence of the cerebrum as to play a relatively small part in binocular vision. Their most important rôle, that of rotating the eyes against inclinations of the head so as to tend to stabilise the vertical meridian, has already been noted. In addition, they clearly contribute to the maintaining the steady position of the eyes in spite of body movements. The overriding importance of occipital impulses is, however, amply demonstrated by the fact that not only does destruction of both labyrinths entail no loss of eye movements, except torsions, but that the eyes and cortex can, in man and the primates, take over the primary duty of the labyrinths, namely the stabilizing of body posture.

As we have already seen, the work of Holmes and others has located the pontine centre for conjugate lateral gaze in the immediate neighbourhood of the vestibular nucleus, if not in it. The issue is somewhat complicated by the large size of this nucleus, the fact that it is somewhat arbitrarily split up into four portions, the nucleus of Bechterow, the triangular nucleus, the nucleus of Deiter and the nucleus of Roller; in addition, its boundaries are not all well defined and its various connections are far from having been completely worked out. The present knowledge is clearly summarised by Duke-Elder (49). In view of the fact that there are three pairs of semi-circular canals in three planes, and that there are three extra-ocular muscle planes, many attempts have been made to associate individual canals with individual muscle planes. No such scheme has ever had any general acceptance and de Kleyn (77) and others have shown evidence that each semi-circular canal exerts some influence on all three muscle groups.

Even though the labyrinthine reactions do not appear to be of great importance for our immediate purposes, they are of great value clinically for the assistance they give in the localization of lesions and verifying that central pathways are intact. Anyone old enough to have danced an old-time waltz, who is unacquainted with the subjective symptoms of vestibular nystagmus should lose no time in seeking medical advice if he has not already done so.

The cerebellum is the head ganglion of the proprioceptive system, of which the labyrinths, as the chief proprioceptive organs of the head, are the most important element. Sherrington (125) has shown that the cerebellum is a purely motor organ whose function is the maintenance of the tone of the voluntary motor system so that it is always in a state of readiness; it maintains the equilibrium of the organism but takes no part in the execution of movements. Walshe (142) describes decerebrate rigidity as an exaggeration of normal postural tone, in which extensor tone in particular is exaggerated. He points out that it is produced by the ablation of the cerebrum and continues if the cerebellum is subsequently removed. On the other hand, the ablation of the cerebellum alone does not lead to decerebrate rigidity but the subsequent ablation of the cerebrum does. Spinal transection below the level of the superior colliculi abolishes it. He describes the function of the cerebellum as the integration of the postural with the phasic elements of motor activity. The cerebellum is necessary for the voluntary activation of these reflexes and the cerebrum acts on them via the cerebellum and not vice-versa. In this reflex co-ordination Rademaker (quoted by Duke-Elder) considered the red nucleus to be the main centre for the distribution of muscle tone and the righting reflexes that control posture. This, as he points out, is not universally accepted. Since the fibres of the third nerve pass through it any lesion of this nucleus is likely to cause oculo-motor involvement.

We have made no mention of proprioceptive impulses "fed back" from the extraocular muscles themselves, for the reason that, though the point may not be finally settled, it seems to the writer to be clearly established that, normally, little or no use is made by the central nervous system of any proprioceptive impulses from the extraocular muscles. This point will be considered along with the histology of the muscles.

There is no need to describe the course and connections of the nerves innervating the extraocular muscles, or the mechanics and macroscopic anatomy of those muscles in a paper of this sort; these points are too well known and agreement on them is complete. They are, however, very remarkable structures, as might be expected from the extreme delicacy of the movements that they are called upon to perform. As Lancaster (30) has pointed out, these muscles are, by analogy with other muscles, large enough to exert a hundred times the traction that is ever called for. In addition, the nerves supplying them are extremely large in comparison to the size of the muscle that they innervate. They are generally described as consisting of coarse medullated and fine non-medullated fibres (Cogan, Wolff, and others). They end in relation to the fibres of the appropriate muscles, these fibres may also be classed as large and small, though there is very considerable variation and the division is not so clear cut as is the case with the nerve fibres.

The two sizes of nerve fibres have been demonstrated conclusively in the muscle proper, though the position is less clear in the trunk of the nerve. The large fibres end in normal motor end plates with from five to twenty such plates in relation to each large muscle fibre. The fine non-medullated fibres end in unusual terminations which have been variously described as clawlike or grapelike. They have been described in the extraocular muscles of all mammals but have not been conclusively demonstrated elsewhere, though Woolard (152) states that there is some reason to suppose that they may be found in the tongue, the muscles of mastication, and of the face, though he adds that further evidence is needed before that statement can be accepted. Similar if not identical terminations have been demonstrated in the skeletal muscles of cold blooded animals (78). These atypical fibres innervate the smaller muscle fibres and are found principally in the insertional third of the muscle. Woolard (152) made a special study to try to establish whether the two forms of innervation overlapped. Any overlapping must be exceptional since he never found the two types of fibre in relation to one muscle fibre, though as he points out, observation alone cannot prove a negative. If the finding of Lockhart and Brandt that all fibres of the human eye muscles run the whole length of the muscle is correct, the reliability of this finding becomes more doubtful (93). Hines (71) did find such overlapping in the rabbit. Both Hines and Woolard state that the majority of these endings are epilemmal, though some were hypolemmal.

Before proceeding to consider the probable origin and function of these fibres, there are two other peculiarities of the extraocular muscles that we should notice; the first is that the amount of elastic tissue, both in the perimysium and septa, is quite abnormally large (150) which probably contributes to the great delicacy of adjustment that they can achieve; a point to which we will recur when we come to consider fixation. The other peculiarity of these muscles is that, according to Duke-Elder (48), they are the only muscles of the body which give a prolonged tonic contraction to acetylcholine without being denervated; a property which they have in common with the skeletal muscles of many cold blooded animals.

These fibres have been assigned to various sources and functions. The suggestion that they belong to the cervical sympathetic is ruled out by the work of Woolard (152) and Corbin and Oliver (44), who found that the complete removal of as much as possible of the cervical sympathetic trunk including the superior cervical ganglion had no effect on these terminations. Woolard and also Hines (71) found that these endings degenerated in the appropriate muscles if the third nerve was divided as close to the brain stem as possible. Hines reported that the only endings that survived were those in relation to blood vessels. Nicholson (107) has reported isolated ganglion cells near the root of the third nerve. These could be members of the cranial autonomic system stranded in their peripheral migration, but are more probably sensory, and Tozer and Sherrington (130) found that almost twenty fibres survived in the monkey, the cat, and the rabbit after the sixth nerve had been cut, but they were far too few to play the important part of proprioception normally ascribed to these fibres, or to correspond with the many fine fibres actually found in the muscles. Sherrington has shown that from a third to a half of the nerve fibres to limb muscles are sensory (126). These few cells might also be vestiges of the somatic sensory ganglion associated with the nerves which disappear more or less completely during development.

Woolard has shown that the number of fine fibres in the trunks of the oculo-motor nerves is not nearly enough to account for those found in the extraocular muscles, and that these fine fibres are almost certainly the result of the branching of fibres which are medullated in the nerve trunks, and which lose their myelin sheaths when nearing their destination. Believing them to be the sensory supply of the muscles, he suggested that their origin would prove to be the mesencephalic root of the fifth nerve and that confirmation of this hypothesis would be proof of their sensory function. Unfortunately, the converse is not true; the fact that it has been shown since that they do not come from this root of the fifth nerve is no real proof that they are not sensory.

Corbin and Oliver (44) found no degeneration of these fibres or their terminations in the cat after the cell content of the mesencephalic root of the fifth nerve had been completely destroyed. Destruction of any part of the large celled motor areas of the nucleus of the third nerve always led to such degeneration. They therefore concluded that the cells of origin of these atypical fibres were in, or very close to, the nuclei containing the cells of the normal motor fibres. Woolard had already shown they did not originate from either the Edinger-Westphal nuclei, or those of Darkschewitch.

Following up this work with Harrison, Corbin (43) found that electro-stimulation of the peripheral end of the third nerve gave rise to action currents in the third nerve nucleus and in the intra-medullary part of the third nerve, but nowhere else in the brain stem. Despite their own and other work, Corbin and Oliver also believed these atypical fibres to be sensory. The work of Hines and of Tozer and Sherrington makes it very unlikely that the fifth nerve serves sensation in the fibres of the extra ocular muscles.

Wilkinson (147), who made an extended study of these terminations, particularly in lizards and snakes, came to the conclusion that in these animals many of these terminations, if not most, were hypolemmal and probably immature motor end plates. The epilemmal ones would presumably be immature sensory terminations. Wilkinson found that many muscle fibres received both forms of innervation in reptilia. Woolard, ten years later, made a special study of mammalian material, as already quoted, to clear this point and found no overlapping. Woolard thought that the majority of these terminations were epilemmal, but this is a notoriously difficult point to settle. Wilkinson's modified teasing technique yielded particularly convincing microphotographs demonstrating hypolemmal terminations in his material with a proportion of epilemmal, but his material contained normal sensory terminations as well and he regarded both the hypolemmal and the epilemmal forms as immature variants.

The writer has attempted to use Wilkinson's technique on a fragment of inferior oblique from a myectomy. His preparations were not good enough to yield decent photographs but the best slides seemed to show that in man most of these terminations were hypolemmal and so, presumably, motor terminations. Professor Lovatt Evans shares this view (56).

Wolff (150) shows a microphotograph of a typical muscle spindle, such as is associated with proprioception in other parts of the body in a human rectus muscle. This was the first instance that the writer knew of, though Buzzard recorded one as long ago as 1908 (24). The author is indebted to Mr. Wolff for having called his attention to the work of Cooper and Daniel which appeared after he had written the chapter and which compels reconsideration of the whole question of proprioception in the human extraocular muscles (41).

These workers have found as many as forty-seven muscle spindles in a human inferior rectus muscle. This being about the same number as is found in the first lumbrical muscle of the human hand, a muscle of about the same length which is undoubtedly endowed with proprioception. They found such muscle spindles in all the extraocular muscles and though they did not make a detailed investigation of their relative frequency in the different muscles, they say that they appear to be most numerous in the inferior rectus with the other recti following, somewhat fewer in the obliques, and rare in the levator.

The reason for these structures having escaped notice for so long, despite the repeated searches that have been made for them, must lie in the fact that their capsules are far more delicate and more difficult to demonstrate than those of the muscle spindles of human skeletal muscles, and the authors compare them to the description of the muscles spindles of the human fœtus given by Forster and Cuajunco (60) (45), and suggest that this may indicate that they are a primitive form, just as Wilkinson suggested that the grapelike nerve endings were a primitive form.

These same workers have, in collaboration with Whitteridge, recorded afferent discharges with the stereotoxic technique and the needle electrode in the oculomotor nuclei when the detached extraocular muscles of a goat were pulled (42).

These workers appear to consider that proprioception plays an essential part in the posture of the eyes. The writer certainly feels that their findings are the most formidable evidence that those who do not believe this must answer.

We have seen that the nerve supply to the extraocular muscles is enormously greater than that to any other muscle of comparable size, and that the delicacy of the adjustments that they have to make is far greater than those required, even from the muscles of the hand. If proprioception played thc important part in eye posture that it does in skeletal posture one would surely expect that the number of stretch receptors would bear much the same proportion to the total innervation as it does elsewhere. As we have seen, the number of receptors found is of the same order as that found in other muscles of its own size but not provided with its own innervation.

Cooper and Daniel have drawn attention to the fact that these receptors have been demonstrated in the eye muscle of members of the Ungulata with high centres of gravity which are noted for their sure-footedness, such as goats and deer, but they are also found in pigs and sheep. None of these animals has a fovea so they do not need the more delicate adjustments of the line of sight necessary for human binocular vision. It does seem likely that good postural control of the eyes from proprioception from neck and other skeletal muscles is of far greater importance to them than to man, in whom such control is difficult to demonstrate. Against this must be mentioned that such control is easy to demonstrate in the rabbit, while muscle spindles have not been found in its extraocular muscles. However, when we remember the length of time for which their existence in man has been denied, we have to admit that they may yet be found.

Cooper and Daniel have also called attention to the fact that undue manipulation of the eye muscles during an operation may cause nausea to the patient, and suggest that this may be evidence of proprioception. It seems to the writer to be more convincing as evidence against proprioception. The mind's knowledge of the position of the eyes is what keeps our surroundings fixed when the eyes move and it seems more probable that the nausea is due to the movement of the patient's surroundings due to the passive movements of the eye of which the brain has no knowledge.

In view of the fact that muscle spindles were demonstrated in the eye muscles of Ungulata long before they were found in man, it seems reasonable to suppose that their capsules are thicker in these species. Cooper and Daniel do not mention the point, or reproduce microphotographs from animal material and comparison of microphotographs from different laboratories is unsatisfactory so, though other papers make it seem probable, we cannot state this as a fact. It accords well with their suggestion that in the human these structures may be a primitive form, though it seems equally probable that they may be a degenerate form. An alternative suggestion that they make is that the thicker capsule of the skeletal stretch receptors may be for protection which is not needed in the orbit, but this would apply equally to other mammals.

The writer is, therefore, inclined to believe that these spindles played a part in stabilising the eyes when man was getting onto his feet, not too securely at first, but that their function is now largely lost. The fact that they seem to be most numerous in the inferior rectus may support this suggestion and their presence there might be the explanation of Bielchowsky's dissociated vertical divergence.

It is natural to ask why such immature and primitive structures should survive in the extraocular muscles and probably nowhere else. The writer thinks that the answer must lie in their great antiquity and stability. The single median eye of Daphnia, a composite eye made up of a number of ommatidia, has four recti muscles which are very similar to those of the vertebrate, and the four recti and two obliques are universal among vertebrates. Atwood (7) considers that they are derived from the first three myotomes of the embryo. In the human embryo the primitive mass from which the extraocular muscles develop has divided into separate muscles, and all three nerves have reached it by the fifth week (about 9 mm.). No other muscles can show so long a history almost without change, so it ought not to surprise us if they retain certain primitive features.

It seems to me that the only grounds for regarding the fibres with the grape or clawlike endings as sensory are that they are atypical and that there are no others adequate to provide for the fine proprioceptive sense which has been assumed for the extraocular muscles. The evidence seems to me overwhelming against the existence of any such proprioceptive sense and there seems to be positive evidence to suggest that, however atypical, these fibres are in fact motor fibres; they are the only fibres known to innervate a considerable proportion of the muscle fibres; they arise, almost certainly, in a motor nucleus, and it is difficult not to associate them with the sensitivity of these muscles to cholinergic drugs which produces a motor effect. These points would not be enough to carry conviction if a well developed proprioceptive sense had ever been demonstrated in the extraocular muscles, but no such sense has been demonstrated and the writer hopes to show later that such a proprioceptive sense would be a hindrance to binocular vision.

Against the assumption of this proprioceptive sense we have the fact that stretching individual eye muscles results in pain, but in no sense of the eye having turned, and that it does not give rise to action potentials in their nerves (38) such as Cooper, Daniel and Whitteridge recorded in the goat. Passive movements of the eyes lead to the sensation that the subject's environment has moved, as also will movement in response to reflexes from a sufficiently low level; for example, the giddiness resulting from rotational nystagmus. Similarly, if the eye fails to move in response to an innervation the environment seems to move; this is found in cases of recent paralysis and when an anæsthetized eye is prevented from performing a voluntary movement. Still more striking evidence of the absence of any proprioception of the position of the eyes is afforded by the records of autokinetic movements made by the Royal Air Force medical team working under Air Commodore (now Air Vice-Marshal) P. C. Livingstone, whereby a dim light in an otherwise dark room may appear to move as much as twenty degrees when, in fact, the light was fixed and the subject's eyes have moved without his knowledge.

It seems, then, to be clearly established that there is no true proprioception in the extraocular muscles and that the sensory fibres from the fifth nerve which accompany the blood vessels are sufficient to account for the sensations of pain, which appear to be the only sensations which can be evoked in them. If this is conceded there is no need to postulate a sensory rôle for the atypical fibres in the face of the evidence which suggests a motor rôle for them; a view that Woolard seemed to incline to in 1937 (153).

The only other structure which can contribute to our appreciation of depth is the ciliary muscle, and a few workers have suggested that proprioception of accommodation plays a part in our judgment of distance. This seems very unlikely on many grounds. One-eyed subjects acquire the trick of moving their heads to obtain a parallax of motion so quickly, and until they acquire it their distance judgment is so poor as to make it seem unlikely that they possess any useful alternative.

Fincham and Adamson's (1) work on the association of accommodation and convergence shows that the eye has a very considerable depth of focus, especially, of course, in bright light, and it also suggests that the accommodation moves in discontinuous jumps. Fincham's theory of accommodation (57) is now generally accepted everywhere and it describes a mechanism whereby the contraction of the muscles releases the pull of the zonule on the capsule of the lens, thereby permitting this structure to mould the plastic lens to a different shape. The only stimulus for a change of accommodation is the blur circle, or other aberration pattern on the retina, and there is no provision for the organism to know whether a given blur circle is the result of rays that have already crossed, or of uncrossed rays, other than trial and error. Such a mechanism hardly calls for serious consideration as a factor in anything so sensitive as our perception of depth.

Classically the ciliary muscle is described as being in three portions, the meridial, radial, and circular. Brucke named the meridional position the tensor choroideæ, though, as Duke-Elder points out, it is an improbable function for any muscle. It has generally been considered as exerting a pumping action on the canal of Schlemm, though this is questioned by Wolff. The radial and circular portions of the muscle are continuous and inseparable, though the meridional fibres are commonly called Brucke's muscle, while the radial are sometimes called Muller's muscle; neither name rests on good historical grounds. Fincham's work suggests that the whole muscle should be considered one and that there is a continuous transition from the meridional to the radial fibres. The writer's observations bear this out.

There has been considerable controversy on the innervation of this muscle complex for a long time. That the main innervation is parasympathetic is obvious from the fact that it is paralysed by atropine. The parasympathetic, or cranial autonomic outflow acts, in general, in opposition to the true sympathetic system. Both are integral parts of the central nervous system, but they have migrated outwards, sometimes so far that their cell stations are in the peripheral organ concerned. It is generally accepted that the ciliary muscle is innervated by fibres from the parasympathetic, or cranial, autonomic system relaying in the ciliary ganglion. These also innervate the sphincter pupillæ. The dilator pupillæ is innervated by sympathetic fibres from the superior gervical ganglion which reach the orbit by way of the carotid plexes, the Gasserian ganglion, the ophthalmic division of the fifth nerve, and the long ciliary nerves.

There has been an acute controversy ever since histology became a science as to whether there was a dual innervation to the ciliary muscle, such as has been demonstrated in the iris. The two situations are similar and the histological picture gives plenty of room for personal convictions. The long ciliary nerves run forward in the scleral wall, frequently, at least, leading to groups of cells, the accessory episcleral ciliary ganglia, from which fine branches pass (Agababow, quoted by Duke-Elder) to many structures including the ciliary body. Duke-Elder gives a very clear statement of the position of our knowledge on the subject up to about 1928 and sums up in favour of the conclusion that the true sympathetic system plays no part in accommodation. Recently the question has been reopened by various workers, the most important observation being that of Matteuci (100) who claims to have demonstrated, by the method of Gros, sympathetic as well as parasympathetic fibres both in the radial and circular portions of the muscle. The work of Moreu (104) also seems to support the theory of a dual innervation.

The whole question is still open for discussion, but it is perhaps safe to regard the sympathetic influence as not much more than a second-order effect and agree with Duke-Elder to regard the parasympathetic system as the only important innervation for accommodation. In the same way, it is probably safe to ignore the humoral control of eye muscles. It is quite possible, even probable, that some humoral mechanism plays a part in the control of the intraocular muscles, and even of the extra-ocular, in view of their cholinergic sensitivity, but if so it must act too slowly to be important to us in our present study.

I cannot resist the temptation to conclude this chapter with Duke-Elder's translation of Claude Bernard's description of the autonomic nervous system: " It is as though Nature thought it prudent to remove the important phenomena which it controls from the caprice of an ignorant will."

CHAPTER II

VISUAL REFLEXES

It is obvious that a two-neuron reflex arc is theoretically possible and it is likely that such exist in the human body, though probably not in the simplest possible form, of a receptor activating an effector with no other control of the effector, but it is certain that no such simple reflex plays any part in binocular vision. The blink reflex in response to a threat must be one of the oldest and most unconditional of all the eye reflexes; it is also one of the quickest acting, yet the work of Rademaker and ter Braak (115) makes it clear that the impulse leading to the closing of the lids must pass through both the occipital and the parietal cortex on its way to the seventh nerve, which it probably joins as fibres from the third nerve nucleus to innervate the orbicularis muscle. When we remember that it is almost certain that there are no direct communication fibres from the occipital cortex to the parietal, and that all visual fibres have made two synapses in the retina and another in the lateral geniculate before they arrive at the cortex, it becomes clear that the minimum possible path for the blink reflex is one of eight elements and that the path is probably longer still.

This elaborate mechanism serves the oldest and most imperative of all the ocular reflexes, for it is on this reflex that the integrity of the eye depends. Moreover, it must be quick acting if it is to serve its purpose. It does serve its purpose remarkably well; many a time have the writer's eyelids closed in time to catch a particle of brass flying from the edge of the cutting tool of a lathe running at over a thousand revs a minute.

This imperative purpose could be served more quickly by a shorter neuron chain, and it is reasonable to ask whether it would not be better served by a shortened private pathway, say, via the colliculi direct to the third nerve nuclei. Moreover, it is a simple reflex in that there is only one response involved. Yet such an arrangement would be useless for any but the most primitive creature, whose eyes did little more than serve a simple purpose such as phototropism, as every significant change in illumination, and that implies every useful message, would lead to the creature's eyes closing. For a blink reflex to be useful to the higher animals, it must be initiated at a level capable of discriminating between a harmless signal and a threat.

The blink reflex has been dealt with at some length because it is simple, of great antiquity and necessarily a rapid one. Yet, as we have seen, it needs quite an elaborate neural mechanism if it is to serve its purpose. We must not expect that the pathways involved in the higher reflexes will be so simple or that they will be known with any accuracy. It is not even possible to list them for authorities differ greatly in the number of distinct ones that they recognise, and the distribution that they claim for them in the animal world. Chavasse (36) claims that all vertebrates have binocular vision and goes so far as to state that " purely monocular movement, even in response to a purely monocular stimulus, does not occur in the vertebrate series ". He even goes on to state that the often observed monocular movements of a chameleon are the result of the cancelling out of a vergence with a version for one eye. This opinion is in direct contradiction to that of Rochon-Duvigneand who has made a most extensive study of the ocular movements of the lower vertebrates and has come to the conclusion that most ocular movements in fishes and many in reptiles are truly monocular. The writer, on the other hand, has repeatedly observed conjugate binocular movements by tropical fish in an aquarium but he has yet to see a definite monocular movement.

Chavasse regarded the " Binoculus " as the common heritage of the whole of the vertebrates. A study of the available literature seems to make this view untenable. That some fishes, birds and reptiles possess a form of stereopsis by proprioception of convergence seems certain. Many birds of prey possess, in addition to the highly differentiated lateral fovea which serves their very acute distant vision, a second temporal fovea in the centre of the binocular field of each retina which might easily serve a crude convergence stereopsis. Rochon-Duvigneand's description of a chameleon bringing his second eye to bear on an insect already fixated by one eye before shooting out its tongue to catch it seems to argue some stereoscopic sense, though he quotes a record, that the writer has not been able to verify, of a chameleon which had lost one eye and yet retained its skill as a catcher of flies. Among the fishes the most remarkable example of visual skill is the Archer Fish, Toxotes, who can bring down a fly with almost 100 per cent accuracy at three to four feet by projecting a jet of water from just below the surface. In view of the fact that apparent direction is changed by refraction at the surface and that the jet of water must have a curved trajectory due to the effects of gravity, it seems to the writer impossible to doubt that this creature has some form of stereopsis.

These examples seem to suggest strongly that there are birds, fishes and reptiles which possess a form of binocular vision which gives them a measure of stereopsis. This does imply that representatives of each of these classes of vertebrates possess the power of bifixation with in some cases, at least, proprioception of convergence; but this is a very long way from claiming a binoculus for them and stereoscopic vision such as is inferred in the higher mammals and demonstrable only in man.

The evidence of comparative anatomy is against the existence of binocular vision such as we know in any class below the mammals, and it seems probable that it does not appear among them except in a comparatively few higher types. Only the mammals above the Monotremes and Marsupials have an incomplete crossing in the chiasma, so it is only among the placental mammals that the right and left hand portions of the fields of the two eyes are brought together in the cerebrum, a condition which appears necessary for the development of a binoculus. Even among the lower orders of mammals there are very few uncrossed fibres and the most direct objective evidence of binocular vision, the consensual pupil reaction, can be elicited only in three orders, the Carnivora, the Pinnipedæ, and the Primates.

The fixation reflex is by far the most important from the point of view of this study. It has been subdivided into different elements by Chavasse and others, but the phase which interests us is that which Chavasse calls the refixation reflex. The most primitive visual reflexes were those which kept the eyes directed to the same point despite the movements of the head and body. As we have seen, they can still be elicited in man, but with the increased refinement of his fixation they have grown progressively less important.

Though this is a study of binocular vision, it is logical to start with a consideration of monocular fixation. It used to be taught that the eyes performed continuous fine nystagmoid movements over the retinal mosaic. The purpose of this was assumed to be to avoid fatiguing individual retinal receptors. Hering suggested that this " dither " might serve to increase the resolving power of the eye by some scanning process, though the writer must admit to a complete inability to see how it could fail to have the opposite effect.

The most carefully controlled objective investigations are those of Lord and Wright (94, 94a). These workers find a continuous fine tremor with occasional larger kicks of about ten minutes of arc, after which the eye seems to take up a slightly different fixation. They also show evidence that these kicks may correlate with the pulse. If this is so it is likely that the new fixation that the eye appears to take up is, in fact, a change of position of the eye in its orbit. The problem of recording the movements of the eye during steady fixation by objective means is seriously complicated by the fact that the eye is not fixed in its orbit but is loosely slung; it can shift its position laterally by quite gross amounts and can be moved sideways by digital pressure by as much as three millimetres while maintaining fixation. A further possible source of error in these recordings is that, in the interests of better head fixation, these workers had their subject lying down and looking vertically upwards. Unfortunately this position is one in which the eye is not supported by the thickened portion of Tenon's capsule, known as the ligament of Lockwood, but rests almost directly on the semi-fluid orbital fat from which it is separated by the extremely thin posterior part of the capsule while gravity is acting in a direction which is not normal during precise fixation.

Hartridge and Thompson (69) have also studied this question with an objective technique and do not find nearly such large fixation movements as these. The author's observation (33), that visual acuity is substantially less in the prone position than in the erect, seems to indicate that it is the prone position that is responsible for part of the eye movements recorded by Lord and Wright.

The subjective investigation of the question is just as difficult. It is easy for an observer to satisfy himself that he can maintain fixation on either of two dots whose centres are one minute of arc apart, and change fixation from one to the other at will, provided that his acuity is good enough to resolve them. This does not prove, even to the observer, that his fixation has not changed but only that any change that has occurred has been allowed for by the brain. The most convincing subjective evidence yet published is that of Hartridge (67) who discovered with the micro-stimulator a small group of red-blind cones subtending well under a minute in the fovea of his own left eye, and found that he could maintain fixation on a neighbouring white target while a red stimulus remained invisible since it fell on this red blind area. He was even able to use this group of red blind cones as a reference point in order to locate his fixation points for stimuli of different colours.

If we do not accept the proposition that the eye can maintain fixation to within one minute of arc for a few seconds at least, we are compelled to believe that there is a proprioceptive mechanism capable of providing the necessary data to enable the brain to allow for movements as small as this (0·003 mm. at the surface of the globe or in the length of the muscle, less than 0·01 per cent of its length), and that in muscles which appear to be almost totally lacking in proprioception. The alternative is that these movements are centrally innervated and the red-blind spot and the different colour fixation points observed by Hartridge are cortical and not retinal.

Whatever we choose to believe on these points, we are left with the fact that the eye can turn to a new object of attention and steady on it in a remarkably short time and with very little overshooting or oscillation about its new position. It can also follow a slowly moving object with great accuracy. The dynamics of such problems became the subject of much intensive research during the war as the difficulties of training personnel forced the nations to develop radar sets which would " lock-on " to a target and follow it smoothly without more assistance from a human operator than directing the equipment so that the target was fairly in its field of vision. The ability to do this clearly implies the ability to maintain fixation on a stationary target. The problems involved in the design of such equipment, and also equipment such as gyro-pilots, involved the opening up of a new branch of technology, arising out of what is commonly called communication engineering, which has been aptly named cybernetics in America, the word being derived from the Greek χυβερνήτης, a steersman; the English word governor being derived from a Latin corruption of the Greek word.

This branch of science deals with control mechanisms in general. In its simplest form such a system consists of a receptor and an effector, for instance, the thermometer operated contact and the heating element of a thermostat, a two-neuron reflex arc. So simple a system will always overshoot its mark and the temperature, in this example, will vary by some given amount about a mean value. Even in this simplest possible system, we see the first requirement of a control system, that is what electrical engineers call " feed back ", some portion of the output is fed back to the controlling mechanism.

All these considerations are implicit in " The Integrative Action of the Nervous System ", which Sherrington wrote as long ago as 1906. The treatment of these questions as problems in statistical mechanics is largely the conception of Norbert Wiener, Professor of Mathematics at the Massachusetts Institute of Technology, and his co-workers from other spheres of learning, notably Dr. Arturo Rosenblueth of the Instituto Nacional de Cardiologia of Mexico, formerly of the Harvard Medical School. The principles are set out with their formal mathematical treatment in Wiener's book, *Cybernetics* (145). The conception of proprioception as a feed-back is not new to those of us who were on the " Servo Panel " during the war, where problems of control mechanism design with particular application to the characteristics of the human operator were discussed, but this book marks a great advance in their systematization and application. Wiener and Rosenblueth have already done some most interesting work on heart flutter and fibrillation along these lines (146).

Proprioception does not only report the positions of the limbs to the brain; it is a true feed-back to the controlling mechanism, in that the knowledge of how far short the limb is from the desired position is used to regulate the velocity with which it is moving. Anyone who has found one less step than he expected when walking down stairs knows how fast his foot is moving nine inches before it reaches its intended destination from the jar with which it meets the floor. This is an example of a true feed-back and clinical evidence shows that its utilization is a function of the cerebellum. Unlike the case of the simple on and off thermostat, here it is the velocity of approach which seems to be related to the distance yet to go. Such a system is capable, under suitable conditions, of performing its task without overshooting and going into oscillation, and it is a mechanism of this sort which maintains the stable and dynamic posture of the body, a pure reporting mechanism, such as the word proprioception as opposed to kinæsthetic might imply, would go out of action when the erect posture was achieved leaving the body in neutral equilibrium ready to fall on the least disturbance.

A very brief and non-mathematical consideration of the possible characteristics of a feed-back system seems worth while, but those who want a formal treatment of the subject should refer to a standard work, such as " Servomechanisms " by McColl (101) or to Turing (132) for details of the application of mathematics to the nervous system. Every system that involves movement must possess inertia and as a consequence on and off mechanism controlled by a simple feed-back must oscillate. If we proceed to the next stage where the velocity of movement is controlled so as to be proportional to the displacement from the desired position, we should be in the position of Achilles who is reported never to have quite caught up with the tortoise. Such a system generates a curve of pursuit which lies wholly within the generating curve. It will not oscillate so long as the conditions are such that its output velocity is truly proportional to displacement, but here again, inertia and other factors are likely to prevent this condition from being realised. If so, it may oscillate but it is quite possible that the oscillations will be small and the resultant motion preferable to the true pursuit curve. The important point to notice is that a feed-back system may be stable in that it executes small oscillations about the desired point, or it can be an unstable one which if it once goes into oscillation will do so uncontrollably. The criteria are mathematical and unnecessary for our present purpose.

That a system controlled by a feed-back mechanism must have one definite objective, unless it is designed to generate oscillations, is so obvious as to need no discussion. It follows that one single quantity must be used as the basis of the feed-back, though more than one derivative may be used. If information is fed back from two sources they must, clearly, feed back the same information if the system is to be stable, in which case one of them becomes redundant and lowers the reliability of the system, in that any misalignment will tend to lead to oscillation. Since fixation is necessarily controlled by the displacement of the object of attention from the desired fixation point it seems clear that in an animal with a highly differentiated fovea a true kinæsthetic sense in the extra-ocular muscles would be a handicap rather than a help; there is therefore no need to postulate such a sense or to assume that there are nerve terminations to serve it.

If the objective of a feed-back system is ill-defined in comparison with the sensitivity of the system, it is bound to oscillate. This is what occurs in the nystagmus that accompanies congenital maldevelopment of the macula and which is commonly seen in cases where congenital cataracts have been operated on after infancy.

Although bi-fixation is an essential to normal fusion, the fusion reflex cannot be regarded as nothing more than two fixation reflexes acting together. As we saw in the last chapter, Bielchowsky, unlike Chavasse, regarded the fusion reflex as the only true oculo-motor reflex, in that it is the only one which operates wholly below the level of consciousness and is altogether beyond the reach of the will. Fixation is a voluntary function, but Burian (23) has shown that suitable peripheral stimuli can often be fused while central fusion is still impossible, and furthermore that peripheral stimuli can break central fusion even though the subject is concentrating on the central target. This observation has been confirmed by Winkleman (149).

Because the process of encephalisation has brought them within the reach of the will, Bielchowsky (16) did not regard the accommodation-convergence reflexes as pure reflexes. It seems, however, wiser to agree with Chavasse in treating them as such, at any rate during the development period.

Chavasse recognised three reflexes which he called accommodation reflexes, though he considered that they were all three built on an older convergence reflex.

1. The Occipital Accommodation Reflex, which he considered to be inborn and to produce an amount of accommodation properly appropriate to the convergence being exercised. It seems to assume emmetropia and full power of accommodation.

2. The Harmonic Accommodation Reflex whose function is to adjust the accommodation so as to focus the object fixated clearly. In other words, it performs the adjustments necessary to harmonise the occipital reflex with the actual conditions of the individual. It appears to be of later development than the occipital reflex and its power seems limited at first. Later it becomes conditioned and it is probably this reflex that gives enough flexibility to the accommodation-convergence system to allow it to adapt itself to the changes that occur in the power of accommodation during life.

3. The Frontal Accommodation Reflex. This Chavasse describes as forcing accommodation up to the level required for distinct vision, when

that is demanded and cannot be provided by the other two by acting equally on accommodation and convergence.

This last has the most doubtful claim to be regarded as a reflex in that it is to some extent under the control of the will and is the process by which " mental effort " alters convergence. When this alteration of convergence has been achieved the harmonic reflex may be able to refocus the images. It is the use of the frontal reflex for clear vision that leads to accommodative strabismus in hypermetropia.

This account of the accommodation reflexes differs slightly from that given by Chavasse in that the author believes that the harmonic reflex can act to increase or reduce accommodation, whereas Chavasse only claimed for it that it increased it. Experience with " mental effort " (25) strongly suggests that conscious or voluntary interference with convergence or accommodation acts on both together, and that when such interference leads to fusing two images which were previously separate, re-focussing, if it occurs, is achieved by some process outside voluntary control.

The writer has now seen three cases of alternating strabismus of such early onset (under six months) that no conditioned binocular reflex could ever have become established, yet all three, wearing their corrections showed a normal convergence-accommodation relationship under dissociation conditions, and all three showed no significant phoria if the dissociation was long enough. In none of these three cases could fusion be elicited and in none can binocular vision ever have been established. This seems to him to be overwhelming evidence of the correctness of Chavasse's description of the occipital reflex, the foundation on which the other two act.

It seems then that it is the harmonic reflex which is responsible for clear vision in phoria cases, and that it is this reflex which is frequently described as breadth of fusion or relative accommodation. A purely fusional movement is extremely difficult to demonstrate in the convergent direction. It probably exists but it is masked by the harmonic reflex; it is readily demonstrated in the divergent direction and vertically, as there is no other physiological function that can be confused with it.

This leads to the consideration of muscle balance. A very great many people have endeavoured to define the position of rest of the eyes; their number testifies to the difficulty of the task, as does the fact that no one definition has gained universal acceptance. The fact that these attempts have been so numerous is the author's excuse for adding to their number. Not that he expects to succeed where so many have failed, but that with so many definitions available it seems desirable to leave the reader in no doubt as to what is meant here.

Before attempting to give a definition, it is necessary to clear the ground of various ideas that have been advanced from time to time and which do not seem to serve any useful purpose. The first of these is the " position of anatomical rest ", which must mean either the position assumed by the eyes after death, in which case the question: How long after? seems relevant; or it means the position which the eyes would assume if all the extraocular muscles were denervated. Neither seems very relevant to a discussion of the normal functioning of the binocular apparatus. The next position that has been considered is that assumed in sleep and anæsthesia. We are commonly told that the eyes turn up and out when the subject is asleep, but the evidence for their turning out is very slight, while the turning up is a conjugate movement calculated to provide extra protection, and Bell's phenomenon——the turning up of the eye when an effort is made to close the lids against a resistance—shows that there is a conjugate innervation for this purpose. Anæsthesia provides even more unreliable evidence, as the eyes diverge in the earlier stages but return to what appears to be a parallel position when a deep surgical anæsthesia is reached. The only conclusion that can be drawn safely is that tonus is reduced in muscles innervated by the third and fourth nerves before the lateral recti, innervated by the sixth, are sensibly affected.

The phrase which appeals most to the writer is " the tonic position ", if the word tonic is accepted as meaning the state of minimum innervation which holds the muscles in readiness to act. This condition will be called a state of reflex tonus in deference to those who use the word tonus to indicate the sum total contraction of a muscle at any time.

In an earlier paper the author used the phrase " the natural position of the eyes " (30). This is not a definition, but it does convey what we are attempting to define to anyone who is in fairly close agreement with us; it needs amplification in that it leaves room for every form of quibbling.

We define the position of rest of the eyes " as the mean of their relative positions with one eye fixing a distant object in the primary position when the other has been prevented from fixing for long enough to have assumed the position which it takes up under the influence of reflex innervation alone, and for innervations which are the result of habit, but are not conditioned, to have subsided."

The author is fully alive to many of the objections to this definition; in particular it assumes that all are agreed as to what constitutes reflex innervations and what is meant by non-conditioned habitual innervations, and this point at least must be made clearer. It is characteristic of those tonic innervations which have become incorporated into a conditioned postural reflex that they can be maintained indefinitely without fatigue. It is not unusual to find that when the two eyes of a patient with asthenopic symptoms have been dissociated for long enough, there is a substantial increase in the muscle imbalance recorded which is accompanied by a relief of symptoms. This seems to indicate that parallelism is being maintained by the use of some mechanism above the reflex level and that an innervational state is brought about which is more closely allied to the ciliary spasm of pseudo-myopia than to reflex tonus, and which is resulting in an approximate pseudo-orthophoria. It seems probable that Chavasse's frontal accommodation " reflex " is the mechanism, both of this state and of pseudo-myopia. Further research on this point is in hand.

In the definition proposed above the words: " prevented from fixing long enough . . ." were used. This means Marlow's prolonged occlusion test which has been the subject of a great deal of discussion, some vituperation, and very little research. Marlow's own work was clinical and empirical; and though based on sound reasoning and carried out carefully, the presentation and method of analysis make it very difficult reading. Two facts do emerge from a careful study of his book (99), firstly that occlusion carried out on one eye only revealed a surprisingly high number of hyperphorias, and secondly that even among a group who had been selected because they had asthenopic symptoms a large number showed no significant increase of exophoria.

This test is frequently criticised on the ground that it produces artefacts which have no significance. It is true that occlusion demonstrates Bielchowsky's dissociated vertical divergence (17, 137)—the fact that, in many subjects, either eye will show a moderate degree of hyperphoria after a few days' occlusion. This is a phenomenon commonly associated with rather large vertical fusional reserves, it does not cause symptoms or call for treatment, its only clinical importance is that it makes it essential to give each eye its period of occlusion in order to separate true hyperphoria from dissociated divergence. The point is discussed at some length by Anderson (6).

Though this phenomenon is common it is not universal; the author saw a patient lately who normally showed vertical orthophoria but showed one prism dioptre of right hyperphoria whichever eye was occluded and no change of lateral phoria; the correction of this small error gave her immediate relief from her symptoms.

The other charge against the occlusion test is that it produces large exophorias which have no significance. This appears to be largely based on the fact that a number of patients who complain of asthenopic symptoms have shown much higher exophorias at the end of an occlusion test than they did before. An illogical criticism of a test designed to show this effect, though perhaps less illogical than the complaint, which has also been made, that it has failed to. Marlow (in his book) reported a case where occlusion gave complete relief from symptoms and yet at the end of a long period no phoria was revealed. At that time he expressed the opinion that a longer period would have revealed a phoria; now we should expect to find aniseikonia.

So far as the author knows, Marlow and himself are the only workers who have made day-to-day plots of changing phorias. The results show, after a varying latent period, a typical growth curve which, with small random variations, tends to a steady value which shows no further signs of a change, a result which is quite inconsistent with the assertion which has been made without any evidence to support it, that the longer the period of occlusion the larger the resulting phoria.

Very little has been published on the results of experimental occlusion on subjects selected for normality. In a note published some years ago (27), the author described the findings from a small scale experiment conducted during the war. He feels that the technique used then was inadequate but the work has been repeated on a somewhat larger if still limited scale (32). The results show that certain artefacts are produced by the test. Figures II, 1 and 2, show the mean changes in vertical and lateral phorias for a small group of young adults. The first of these shows very clearly the average amount of dissociated divergence that may be expected, while the second shows the normal increase in exophoria and the drop which occurs when the occluder is changed from one eye

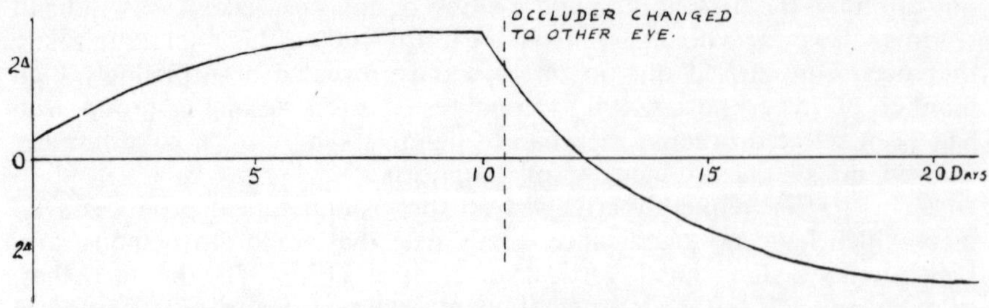

Fig. II. 1. Average Change in Hyperphoria under Occlusion.

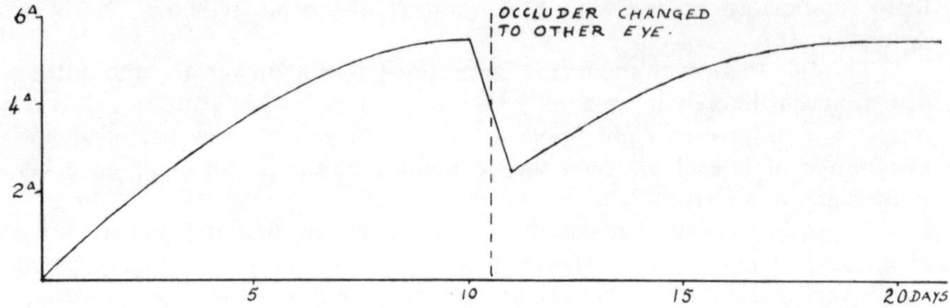

Fig. II. 2. Average Increase in Exophoria under Occlusion.

to the other. This drop shows that the test does produce bigger artefacts than the author formerly supposed, although subsequent experiments seem to show that they are not due to a loss of light tonus. It is remarkably constant both in normal and abnormal cases and it seems likely that it is associated with the vertical divergence.

Another unexpected finding was that almost all subjects developed a considerable amount of excyclophoria, far in excess of normal cyclofusional reserves, yet despite this every normal subject had recovered binocular vision in a matter of seconds. The two abnormal cases are discussed in a later chapter. This also seems to be an artefact of the test and it seems reasonable to suppose that all three effects have the same cause. There is no single muscle whose differential loss of tone could lead to this combination of results; the author therefore tends to the belief that the cause is a differential retention of tonus resulting in an overaction of the inferior oblique.

The author considers that the end result of occluding the two eyes alternately until a steady reading was obtained would be relative position of the eyes under the normal tonic innervations with fusion not operating and the frontal innervation also allowed to subside if necessary. The occipital and harmonic reflexes should be at rest in any case if the subject's refractive error is fully corrected. He believes that in the majority of normal adult subjects this should not differ from the position found by the normal routine with a Maddox rod by more than two or three prism dioptres.

Any heterophoria that is accepted as representing the position of rest is now seen to be the work of the occipital reflex, with fusion frustrated convergence is free and, since the harmonic reflex works on the accommodation only, it should have no action when the accommodation is relaxed. The evidence is that the convergence reflex is of great antiquity, it is certainly demonstrable in all the primates, most of the carnivora and probably in seals. On this, in man at least, is grafted the frontal accommodation reflex and, as we have seen, the combined reflex is inborn and unconditional. Infants converge as soon as they are able to maintain interest in an object for more than the briefest periods. Such an inborn reflex relationship must be approximately the same for everybody, taking no account of individual variations in refraction, which can be large compared to other variations of bodily function. We have seen how this reflex can produce an accommodation-convergence relationship well within normal limits in subjects who have never developed normal binocular vision.

A tightly-linked inborn accommodation-convergence relationship would be adequate for the needs of an animal which did not possess a high visual acuity and had no need of fine vision at its near point, but it is not good enough for man. In order to adjust this occipital reflex to the varying requirements of the individual, man has built on this unconditional reflex the conditioned harmonic reflex. This must be and must remain a conditioned reflex because its function is to give the flexibility necessitated by individual variation to an inborn reflex. It is lacking in infancy and normally formed and consolidated in childhood by the reward of clearer vision which followed regularly on some random change of accommodation innervation. As with other conditioned reflexes, it is in a state of vigorous flux in childhood and becomes progressively less fluid with increasing age. We cannot say at what age this reflex becomes fixed and unalterable. Probably it retains some flexibility into presbyopic age and enables us to adapt ourselves to the changing conditions brought about by the failure of our powers of accommodation. It is on this reflex only that the orthoptist can work, and it is the steady approximation of conditioned reflexes to the fixity of the inborn which sets a limit to the age at which orthoptics can give much help.

The normal process of development in the child is that the extraocular muscles are fully developed and full convergence is available long before the ciliary muscle has developed sufficiently to make enough accommodation for clear near vision possible. The occipital convergence-accommodation reflex is ready but cannot function because one of the muscles under its control is not yet fully differentiated. During the first few months of life clear vision is impossible, not only for lack of the accommodation to focus the near objects which constitute the infant's world and to overcome the normal hypermetropia of early childhood, but the macula is not fully differentiated at birth; yet it is in these first few months that the most vital step is taken and the mind learns that two uniocular images imply one object and the child then learns to fuse these two images into one.

This unification of the two uniocular images and reconciliation of the sense of sight with the sense of touch is the only reward possible at first, and as there is no other to conflict with it binocular vision is normally developed and educated before any of the accommodation reflexes are usable. If, for any reason, this cannot happen, its subsequent achievement is extremely difficult, if not impossible. It is hard enough to learn to do two simple unrelated things simultaneously, let alone two which interact and interfere with each other. It would be interesting to try the effect of the prolonged binocular use of atropine in the attempt to train binocular vision where it had not previously existed.

By the time that the child has developed a useful amount of accommodation fusion should be well enough established to withstand a certain amount of interference, but it is still a new accomplishment, and so easily forgotten if the reward for it is withheld, or some greater reward can be obtained by abandoning it. During this period, when convergence is being exercised without effective accommodation, the inborn occipital accommodation reflex is already trying to act and gradually the object of attention becomes clearer. It is at this stage that the harmonic reflex begins to be built on the foundation of the occipital. It is important to remember that the harmonic reflex is a conditioned reflex, that it is acquired by the individual and is not the heritage of the race. It is for this very reason that it possesses so much flexibility. Because the individual acquires it for himself it is generally adapted to his individual needs and makes allowance for his personal requirements, but being built on an existing reflex there are limits to its power and, moreover, in infancy while the ciliary muscle is still developing and the hypermetropia of childhood is still present the innervation required for clear vision is likely to be greatly in excess of that which will be needed later with the same angle of convergence. As accommodation develops the innervation needed becomes less, less than it was a year ago. This is why esophoria is normal in children. The conditioned reflex is still fluid, the accommodation is, at first, developing and hypermetropia is decreasing while the harmonic reflex is producing the innervation that it learned a little time ago.

We have assumed, so far, that there really is such a thing as relative accommodation and convergence. This assumption is the basis of orthoptics and it is difficult to see how any but a very few fortunate individuals would ever achieve comfortable binocular vision if there were no flexibility in the linkage. Unfortunately, the latest experimental work seems to indicate that if there is any latitude it is exceedingly small and that most of the latitude that has been reported by workers on haploscopes should really be attributed to the depth of focus of the eye. Both Ames and Gliddon (4) working with a modified haploscope and using starpoints of light to measure the accommodative state of the eyes, and Fincham (1), using the coincidence optometer, found that every change in convergence was accompanied by a change in the refraction of the eye.

Yet everyone who has used mental effort to fuse two targets, either by converging or by diverging, has experienced the fusing of the two targets with the accompanying blurring followed after a time by refocussing so that the targets are seen sharply. It is quite impossible to try the experiment on one's self and doubt that after the targets have been fused and the convergence of the eyes has thereby been approximately fixed they can and do change their focus. An unusually intelligent young patient gave the writer recently an extremely vivid description of two targets, fused by over-convergence, coming clear and then slipping back to blurred and finally of holding them single and clear. This is not the description of a depth-of-focus effect and although some retinal slip is probably present in such experiments it cannot be more than a second-order effect.

It looks, at first sight, as if we were confronted with a flat contradiction of the evidence, but Fincham and Adamson, who used subjects ranging in age from 18 to 46, found in each case that the accommodation-convergence relationship had adjusted itself to the changing ocular conditions appropriate to the subject's age. It seems that what these workers and Ames and Gliddon have shown is that in the normal use of the eyes by normal subjects the occipital and the harmonic accommodation reflexes behave as one unconditioned reflex, despite the fact that the latter is a conditioned reflex which retains some flexibility into, at least, late adult life. It is only through the frontal accommodation reflex, if indeed it may be called a reflex, that we can interfere with the harmonic reflex and none of the experiments described by these workers made any call upon it. It may well be that the difficulty of interfering with this reflex is what gives some measure of permanence to orthoptic treatment.

A recent case of the author's seems interesting in this connection. The patient was a girl of fourteen and her objective refraction was R.E. $-1\cdot25$ D sph. $-0\cdot50$ D cyl. 180°; L.E. $-1\cdot00$ D sph. $-0\cdot25$ D cyl. 180°. Muscle balance 2△ esophoria at distance, and 2△ of exophoria at 33 cm. Her unaided vision was R.E. 6/24, L.E. 6/18, the above correction giving 6/5 in each eye. An examination under full atropine cycloplegia seemed desirable, on the chance that she might prove to be a case of pseudo-myopia. Fortunately, this would have been a serious hardship owing to her studies, so we compromised on instilling atropine into the left eye only (1 drop of 1 per cent twice daily for 5 days). In order to spare her the discomforts of uniocular cycloplegia and mydriasis she was told to wear a shade over that eye until the cycloplegia had worn off.

When she came back to be examined under cycloplegia, the refraction of the left eye was found to be $-0\cdot25$ D cyl. 180° only, and that of the right, into which no atropine had been instilled even accidentally as its pupil was not dilated, was found to be $-0\cdot25$ D sph. $-0\cdot50$ D cyl. 180°; each eye read 6/7·5. Her distance muscle balance was then 4△ exophoria.

It seemed obvious that the suspicion that she was a pseudo-myope was well founded and the change in muscle balance suggested the possibility of curing her by orthoptics. Unfortunately nothing could be done immediately as she was returning to school the next day, so, as she was extremely keen on a cure, she was advised to continue using an eye shade for all close work, using her eyes on alternate days and using binocular vision only for games and when out of doors, until the next holidays.

When next seen her exophoria had increased to 6△ at 6 metres and 12△ at near, and her acuity was 6/6 each eye. She was then given adduction exercises by fusing stereo cards by over-convergence and advised to continue monocular reading for another month. Four months later her distance muscle balance was orthophoria, she was emmetropic, and her visual acuity 6/5.

It is impossible to escape the conclusion that her exophoria was anatomical and that it was the cause of the pseudo-myopia and it seems reasonable to suppose that, if left alone, the condition of orthophoria and myopia would have become stable. Since then the author has seen two young myopes show a reduction of about 0·75 D under occlusion together with an increase of exophoria. His own myopia does not show this effect but it seems very possible that it might have done thirty years ago.

This is a picture of what occurs when all goes well, but there is another possibility. The hypermetropia may be greater than normal or the development of the ciliary muscle may be retarded so that the innervation needed for clear vision is well above that which accompanies the convergence necessary for binocular vision. When this occurs the individual has the choice between blurred single vision and clear double vision, as the only means of obtaining clear vision is the frontal intervention which Chavasse called the frontal reflex. Luckily the former choice is the usual one as single vision is generally a greater reward than clear vision; if, however, the blurring is very great the individual may prefer clarity with diplopia. If there is a big difference in quality between the two images, so that one is sharp while the other is not, the risk of the child's accepting diplopia is greatly increased as it is relatively easy, at first, to ignore and then to suppress the poorer image. The result is then a unilateral convergent strabismus with amblyopia of the squinting eye.

Amblyopia arising from suppression has a lot in common with a conditioned reflex, so a few words on the subject may not be out of place at this point. It is a process of cortical inhibition which in process of time requires a fixity which is largely dependent on the age at which it started and the time that it has lasted. It is conditioned, just as is a reflex, by a reward, the same reward that conditions the harmonic convergence reflex: clear single vision. For this reason the usual name amblyopia ex anopsia is objectionable, though it is so well established that it is probably best to accept it. Amblyopia does not appear to be the result of disuse, one myopic eye is seldom amblyopic, provided that it ever had good vision and the general rule is that the less the difference in refractive error between the two eyes, in a unilateral squinter, the deeper the amblyopia. In addition, the prolonged use of a fogging lens or ground glass in the treatment of amblyopia has been said to lead to transferring the amblyopia to the other eye. The author knows of no record of this result following total occlusion.

The suppression in amblyopia is not uniform over the whole field but is selective; the amblyopic eye has just as good peripheral vision as the good eye, while the acuity of the macular area is often depressed to the level of a relatively peripheral part. Later a stage is reached where no one spot in the central area has a higher acuity than its neighbourhood and central fixation is lost. At this stage, when the good eye is occluded the amblyopic eye will make slow, tentative, nystagmoid movements when the patient is asked to fixate a light, for lack of the proper feed-back for fixation. Watchurst (143) finds that in many cases the eye will steady down in a central position if the patient touches the examiner's torch with his finger. This indicates that local sign and its projection may survive fixation. Watchurst considers it a good prognostic sign. At a later stage vision in and round the central area may be suppressed so far as to leave some eccentric spot showing the highest vision that the eye is capable of. This spot then behaves as a false macula or fixation point, though its visual acuity is no greater than that of the corresponding point of a normal eye. What has happened is that the signals from all the more sensitive areas are now inhibited to such a degree that this point has, in effect, the peak sensitivity needed to activate the feed-back system.

I have tried to show, in this and the preceding chapter, that the extraocular muscles have no true proprioception and that no sense of the position of the eyes is fed back to the cortex from the extraocular muscles. Yet that there is something that serves part of the function that such proprioception would is certain. Normally, we know in what direction our eyes are pointing and we make use of knowledge of the degree of convergence of the eyes.

To recapitulate briefly while adding a few more facts, we have, in the dark, no knowledge of passive movements of the eyes and in the light we are conscious of them only by a sensation that the world around us has moved, yet a blind man will often look towards someone who is speaking to him so accurately as to make it difficult to believe that he cannot see, and when we move our own eyes, either voluntarily or through the normal working of any visual reflex, there is no apparent movement of the surrounding scene. An exceedingly rapid voluntary movement of the eyes may give the sensation of some slight movement somewhere, but it is a trifling movement and it seems to be solely the result of deliberately forcing a compensatory mechanism to act at a far greater rate than is normal. Certain eye movements are not compensated for and do result in a sense of movement of one's surroundings, but they do not issue from the normal operation of visual reflexes. The best known is rotation nystagmus which is the result of the gross overloading of a stabilising mechanism. Its effects are well known to almost everyone as giddiness. Less well known but even more easily demonstrated is the apparent movement produced by Bell's phenomenon. The upturning of an eye on closing the lids does not play a part in vision, its function is purely protective and so the compensatory mechanism has no use for the information that the eye has turned and it is not passed to it. As a result, if one attempts to close the eyes against resistance, the only effect is the upturning of the eyes with no compensation in the mind, and the scene appears to move downwards, just as occurs in cases of recent paralysis when the patient attempts to use the paralysed muscle.

If information as to the state of contraction of the extraocular muscles was relayed back from the muscles themselves, there could be no means of discriminating between contractions initiated at different levels, still less could the compensatory mechanism act so as to allow for a movement by a paralysed muscle which had not, in fact, happened. The only alternative explanation is that the innervation to the muscle is repeated to the compensatory mechanism instead of the resulting movement being reported back, presumably in order to avoid interference between two feed-back mechanisms with resulting instability of fixation.

The next question that arises is the level at which this repetition to the cortex of orders to the extraocular muscles operates. So far as the writer knows, the answer is not yet clearly ascertained; however we can say that it must be at some level below the start of the final common path, that is it must be sub-nuclear, otherwise discrimination between innervation of different origins would be impossible. Convergence is the function that seems to throw most light on this question. Most of us are familiar with the way in which a base-in prism tends to make near objects appear larger, or in which two similar objects fused by voluntary divergences seem to enlarge and recede as their separation is increased. When the author first started experimenting on his own binocular vision he could do these tricks very easily; now that he has practised voluntary divergence and dissociating convergence from accommodation to the point that he can fuse stereoscope cards either by over-converging or under-converging with ease, he finds that he can scarcely see the apparent size change at all. Yet, so far as he can tell, any distance judgment that he bases on the state of his convergence is as good as ever. Several friends have said that they find the same. We conclude that each function is reported separately to whatever part of the cortex is responsible for stabilising our impressions of the outside scene.

One point of interest may be mentioned here to complete our discussion of this mental mechanism for compensation for eye movements, even though it belongs to the next chapter and will be dealt with there at some length, and that is that it does not appear to function by making an allowance for the direction in which the eyes are pointing, but by some process which could more accurately be visualized as an adjustment of the local sign of elements of the retina as interpreted by an imaginary median eye. We shall see that it is possible for the mind to project an object that an eye is looking directly towards, in a totally different direction from that in which the eye is directed, if the circumstances are such that that is the easiest reconciliation of conflicting data that it can achieve.

The reader will have noticed that one question, at least, has been directly passed by in silence, that is: What, apart from convergence, is the stimulus to accommodation? The reason for avoiding this question is ignorance. The obvious answer that the error in accommodation remaining when the eyes have converged on the target will always have the same sign will not work, as neither the one-eyed, nor those with two eyes, one occluded, appear to be at all handicapped in focusing; often the contrary seems to be the case. Fincham (58) finds that for small errors of focus, accommodation always moves in the right direction, just as fusional movements are always made in the right direction even though the conscious mind cannot recognise what the direction is. He finds that no effort is made to correct errors of focus if they are large. Ittelson and Ames (75*a*) are investigating the psychological factors affecting accommodation.

Since this chapter was written, a most important paper by Winkelman has appeared (148) in which he describes a series of experiments in which the two eyes were stimulated separately by lights flashing alternately in an apparatus of the haploscope type. The lights were nearly three metres from the subject with a separation of about 1° in one series of experiments, and about 2·4° in another. The layout was such that while each eye saw one light only, the stimulation from the next flash could be made to fall either on the nasal or on the temporal side of the fovea of the other eye.

While the flashing was slow enough the subject experienced the sensation of a single light jumping from side to side; as the frequency of flicker was increased the amount of the apparent jump of the light steadily decreased until, at a certain frequency, the sensation became that of one stationary light; when the frequency of the flashes became high enough to keep the foveæ of the two eyes steadily directed towards their respective lights, so maintaining fusion of the two stimulating lights against the effective phoria resulting from their actual separation. As the speed of flicker was reduced, the same set of sensations was experienced in the reverse order.

The same effects were observed whether the stimulation was bi-temporal or bi-nasal and with both angular separations. The most striking difference noticed was that the reduction of the amplitude of the jump required a higher flicker frequency for bi-temporal stimulation, i.e., convergence, than for bi-nasal. This could be accounted for by a small exophoria that the subject showed, as it was most noticeable for the smaller separation.

If the room was imperfectly darkened, or some other influence interfered with fusion on the lights, the subject still had the sensation of one light jumping about at low frequencies, but as the frequency increased he got the impression of two lights, moving at first but again becoming stationary as the frequency increased. The same effects at about the same frequency were observed if one eye was allowed to see both lights while the other was covered, with little if any difference whether a fixation point was present or not.

These experiments seem to me to prove that stimulation of a peripheral portion of the retina initiates a reflex which tends to bring the object of attention on to the fovea. There is no question of this being the result of a subconscious attempt to fuse separated images of one object as the subject knew that he was seeing separate lights, and this fusion still occurred when one was coloured red and one green. Muscular habit must also be discounted since fusion occurred whether the necessary movement was one of divergence or convergence.

It will be noticed that the maximum apparent movement of the light represents conjunctive movement of the subject's two eyes in order to fix first one light and then the other, while a reduction of amplitude of their movement indicates the start of a disjunctive fusional movement which is complete when all apparent movement ceases.

It is particularly interesting that in all cases the frequency of flicker required to cause all apparent movements to cease varied but little; even in the monocular experiments and the binocular test where other objects prevented fusion of the lights, the jump disappeared at much the same frequency (about 200 per minute). On the other hand, the disjunctive fusional movement always started at a lower frequency when the separation of the targets was $2\frac{1}{2}°$ than when it was $1°$. This is, of course, precisely what one would expect from a stable feed-back system, namely that the greater displacement should lead to the greater righting impulse.

These experiments show clearly that there is a reflex path whose function is to bring the image of objects of attention on to the fovea, and that with binocular stimulation these images will be fused. The writer does not concur entirely with Winkelman's conclusion that there are two reflex paths involved. This is based on the fact that in a room which is not completely darkened the subject first experiences the sensation of one light jumping about, followed, as the frequency increases, by two lights jumping about which finally appear as two steady lights.

In the author's view only one reflex path need be involved, provided that it is capable of being inhibited. That the path is capable of being inhibited is essential to fixation; it is only the object of attention that is fixated and in order to facilitate the reflex path the peripheral object must become the object of attention. A moving object is an object of attention par excellence from the importance to one's ancestors of catching sight both of the animal that they wished to eat and of the one that wished to eat them. Similarly, in a partially darkened room, a flickering light is essentially an object of attention and the eye that sees it will tend to turn towards it, but as the room is not fully darkened there are other objects seen binocularly which will hold fusion and make it easy for the subject to appreciate that there are two flickering lights. Thus the eyes will turn towards each in turn until the frequency of flicker has reached too high a value to operate the fixation reflex. It is not surprising that this value should approximate pretty closely to that which makes steady fusion of two alternately flickering lights possible.

CHAPTER III

THE PHENOMENON OF BINOCULAR VISION

One of the first things that impresses one when one begins to consider binocular vision is its incompleteness. The object of attention is, of course, always seen in single binocular vision and the majority of people pass through life under the vague impression that they have single binocular vision everywhere and at all times, yet most of them have no difficulty in appreciating physiological diplopia once their attention is called to it. Occasionally one encounters people who appear to have binocular vision and yet cannot see it; a certain number of people who have no interest in vision notice it for themselves; and occasionally one encounters a patient whose only trouble is having noticed it and been worried by it.

The importance of physiological diplopia (or introspection diplopia, as it is sometimes and perhaps more aptly called) lies in the light that it throws on the nature of fusion. The existence of such a limitation to one's powers of single binocular vision at once places it in a quite different class of phenomenon to single binaural hearing.

The comparison between these two senses, each furnished with paired organs for distant reception, is of more than passing interest for the warning that it provides against using data from one sense as analogies to illustrate the workings of another. People with good hearing in both ears possess a marked sense of direction for sound which can be embarrassed by interchanging the signals to the two ears with a pseudophone in a somewhat similar way that stereopsis is embarrassed by a pseudoscope. Two loud speakers, one to one's left front and one to one's right front, with similar characteristics in their middle register, one with a good top performance but a weak base, the other reversing these characteristics, will give an astonishing illusion of the orchestra being spread out before one, provided that they are properly phased.

Yet if a signal is fed to one ear only, it is impossible to make a mistake as to which ear heard it, while if the equivalent experiment is tried on the eyes it is impossible by any fair means to tell which eye received the signal. So far as is known, there is no phenomenon in vision to which any phase difference between the stimuli to the two eyes contributes, while the directional effect of sounds appears to be largely dependent on the phase difference between the signals reaching the two ears. Diplopia behind and in front of the object of attention is the rule in vision, even though one image be consistently ignored. No parallel phenomenon is known for the sense of hearing.

The phenomenon of physiological diplopia alone is enough to compel us to reject the suggestion that fusion takes place after projection, and that the mind appreciates the two uniocular images as different aspects of one solid scene, however attractive its simplicity and economy may appear.

The next point that strikes us as we consider this phenomenon is the great facility that the mind has for excluding unwanted signals from consciousness. This suppression is so essential a part of the working of the mind and so well known that there is no excuse for pursuing the point any further, though we shall be compelled to do so later when considering various theories which have been advanced to explain the phenomenon of stereopsis. Let us be grateful that we never hear double.

Diplopia also illustrates projection. It is easy to assure oneself that objects nearer than the point of attention are seen in crossed diplopia while those beyond it are seen in homonymous diplopia. From this it is a step to notice that in relative esotropia we have homonymous diplopia while in relative exotropia we find crossed diplopia. Physiological diplopia is always such as would result from the two uniocular images, each with its appropriate disparities being observed simultaneously by a single cyclopean eye in the median plane.

Normally we have no consciousness of any difference between monocular and binocular projection. Under all natural conditions the differences are small and the discordant elements, which might otherwise call attention to them, are suppressed before they enter consciousness. It is, however, easy to show the difference under artificial conditions. The most dramatic experiment that I know is one devised by the late Alfred Bielchowsky (16), which is illustrated in Figure III 1. R. and L. represent the positions of the subject's two eyes, while O represents a distant object, preferably seen isolated against an indifferent background, such as the sky. P represents a spot on a window pane fairly close to the eyes, placed so that O and P are in line with one of them. H represents a disc with a pinhole held so as to isolate P to the other eye, while N represents a needle held so as to lie on the line of sight to P of this second eye, while the two eyes are converged on P. The mind perceives the three objects N, P and O as being at N′, P and O′ on the straight line C P, C representing a hypothetical median cyclopean eye approximately midway between the two eyes and, we are told, slightly behind them.

The fact that the great majority of people do project from a cyclopean eye has been largely obscured by the conception of the master or dominant eye, which has led to the devising of a number of tests by various workers, the writer included, which were open to the objection that if they answered any question it was the wrong question. The problem is further complicated by the fact that the acuities of the two eyes are often unequal and that most people have a master hand which is very likely to affect the results of some tests.

One worker has advanced the view that, of the two eyes, one gives the line of sight at any given moment, while the other measures the intercept of the object of attention along this line. He goes on to say that, generally, one eye specialises in one rôle and the other in the other task, the line of sight eye being the master eye (55). The writer considers that this theory has now been disproved and mentions it only in case some reader still holds it. He will not deal with it further as he has already dealt with it in a former paper (28). He will, however, deal at some length with the main subject matter of that paper, namely the nature of ocular dominance and the information that the usual tests give.

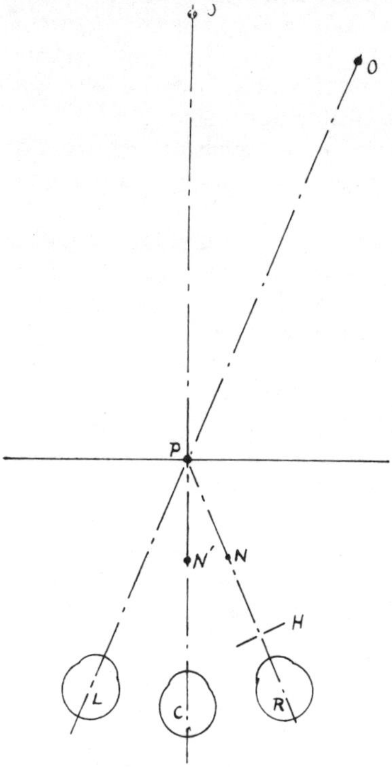

Fig. III. 1.

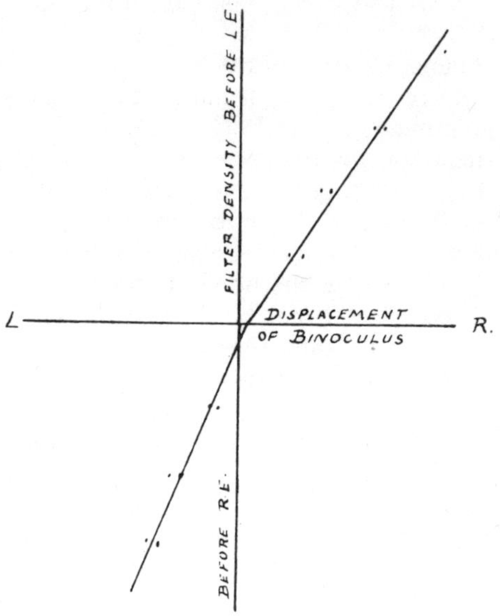

Fig. III. 1A.

The most primitive test is to ask the subject to point at one of the examiner's eyes, without giving any more particular directions. Most people immediately bring up their right hand and align the index fingers between their own right eye and the examiner's eye. The author does, but he finds that if he points with his left hand he aligns it with his left eye, or sometimes between his two eyes, but always nearer to the left. It is clear, as has long been known, that this simple test is at least as much a test of hand dominance as of eye dominance.

It is interesting to compare this apparent change in eye dominance which sometimes accompanies a change of hand with an observation of Watchurst's (143) that an eye which is losing fixation will still fixate the index finger of the homolateral hand, as described in the last chapter, when it is no longer capable of fixating a finger of the other hand.

In the hope of eliminating this ambiguity between hand and eye dominance, various workers have introduced bi-manual tests. One of the best known of these is Parson's manoptoscope. Its essence is that it allows only one eye to fixate the distant test object at a time, for which reason it forces a definite right or left answer on the subject and can give an intermediate answer only in the form of the mean result of several tries. The writer's experience with it is that it selects the eye which first sees the distant object through the aperture; if the acuities of the two eyes are approximately equal, and if this experience is usual, it shows that it is more a test of muscular habit than of eye dominance. Without his correction, the writer is likely to reject the right eye image and choose the left as being the clearer, but this is a process of conscious selection of the better image and, again, no test of ocular dominance.

A test which has had a long run and which has much to recommend it is to give the subject a key ring to be held in both hands and tell him to encircle the distant object with it. It is clear that the use of both hands reduces the effect of hand dominance, but it is equally clear that it cannot eliminate it. As both eyes see the distant object all the time, it is free from some of the objections which can be levelled against the manoptoscope, but it still forces a choice and cannot give a neutral answer. In the writer's experience, it is more consistent in its answers than the manoptoscope, but he is far from being sure that that is not a criticism.

It was in the hope of avoiding some of the sources of error inherent in these tests that he devised the two-handed pointing test that has been taught for some time at the London Refraction Hospital. The subject clasps his two hands together with the index fingers projecting side by side horizontally, and is told to imagine that they are the barrel of a two-handed tommy gun; on the word " fire " he takes a quick shot at the eye that examiner indicates. This test can, and sometimes does, give a neutral answer and quite often gives an answer within the pupil separation, but it, too, is a test of habit in hand and eye co-operation rather than of ocular dominance.

Watchurst (144) has found, over a long series of trials with a test equivalent to the ring test, that in the majority of cases it is the more myopic eye which appears to be the dominant eye. The writer's observations, though on a smaller scale, support him.

Thinking over these results, it occurred to the writer that even in a pointing test physiological diplopia might well force a choice, especially when there was any difference in the refraction of the two eyes. His own habits when shooting with a rifle seem to be relevant at this point. He habitually kept both eyes open, contrary to all army teaching, and fired from his right shoulder. The far point of his right eye lay midway between the sights of the rifle, while his left (about $-0 \cdot 75$ D) could see the target well enough. He did not wear his correction. To the despair of the R.S.M. he was rather a good shot. We know that the diplopic image is normally removed from consciousness, though it remains available for introspection; we also know that suppression does not usually eliminate one entire uniocular image but only such parts as are unwanted. It is obvious that it is preferable to eliminate the less clear image.

Examining tests for ocular dominance with these points in mind, we see that the subject is being asked to pay attention to an object at some metres distance, and to his own hand at about half a metre at one and the same time. When there is any difference of refraction between his two eyes, he can do this by focusing his more hypermetropic (or less myopic) eye on the relatively distant target; the other eye will then have the clearer image of his hand, and it is this image that we expect to be retained in consciousness when one has to be eliminated to avoid diplopia. The more distant target is the primary object of attention and convergence will be directed to it, and the nearer object, his hand, will be imaged on disparate points and require that one image be eliminated.

This seems to suggest a new conception of the dominant eye, namely, it is that eye whose image is retained in consciousness when physiological diplopia requires that one should be removed. We note that this is often the eye which possesses the less clear image of the object of attention, that there is a possibility that the mechanism for the elimination of one image from consciousness may have some connection with the hand in use, and that it is probable that the greater clarity of the image of the nearer object formed by the more myopic eye favours its retention in consciousness. We have also seen that the more myopic eye is the one selected by these tests and, as we know, this turns out to be the right eye more often than chance distribution of errors would lead us to expect. It is generally considered that hand dominance is the result of a leading cerebral hemisphere which will have some anatomical basis, and it is interesting to speculate as to whether this may have any causative influence on the tendency of the right eye to be the more myopic, which is suggested by an analysis of 132 consecutive record cards from the London Refraction Hospital. High myopes and cases of amblyopia were rejected, the average obtained was R.E. 0·32 D more myopic than the left, with a standard deviation of 0·57 D.

An impression formed from work at the Refraction Hospital is that right handed squint patients, with the right eye the more hypermetropic, tend to provide the most intractable cases of amblyopia. There has not yet been time to carry out the necessary work to confirm or disprove this impression and so it is only offered as a speculation. If it proves to be correct it will tend to support the suggestion that there may exist some mechanism for removing from consciousness the image from the eye contralateral to the hand in use, when this removal is advantageous. If this speculation is correct the elimination of the left eye image by a right handed squinter would be, to some extent, a normal physiological function and would not need such active inhibition as the elimination of the image formed by the right eye. Consequently, one would not expect the resulting amblyopia to be so firmly established.

In the article quoted above (28) some experiments designed to demonstrate the point from which the subject projected were reported. Two beads some 40 cm. apart were suspended on fine threads and the subject, with both eyes open, seated about three metres away from them was asked to align himself with them; a plumb bob in the same straight line as the two beads and close in front of the subject was used to indicate the vertical plane in which the centre of projection lay, and the results were recorded photographically. Six consecutive subjects were recorded, the only selection exercised was that they possessed a corrected acuity of not less than 6/6 in each eye. In every case they projected from a point somewhere between the two eyes, though in most cases it proved to be nearer to one eye than to the other.

It was found that if the subject's acuities were noticeably unequal he aligned himself so that the eye with the better distant vision was in line with the beads and that fogging one eye by the addition of + 0·50 D was enough to reverse any bias that he showed. Two cases of low but unequal myopia who habitually went uncorrected aligned themselves to the less myopic eye if uncorrected and almost centrally when corrected. It was also found that placing a neutral filter before either eye would shift the centre of projection towards its fellow.

These results have been criticised by Quick (114) and by Murroughs and Christakos (106) on the grounds that they could observe physiological diplopia under similar conditions. The factors governing physiological diplopia are considered in the next chapter. Francis and Harwood at the London Refraction Hospital (61) have confirmed the author's observations and are extending them on a quantitative basis. Using a more refined technique than the author, they find that, for any given set of conditions, provided that binocular vision does not break down, a good observer will re-align himself to the two targets with an average consistency of at least 2 mm.

Using a photometric wedge to reduce the illumination to one eye at a time, they find that, for some subjects, there is an approximately linear relationship between the reduction of light to the eye and the displacement of the centre of projection, but that the slope of the line is not the same for the two eyes, one eye requiring a greater reduction of illumination for a given shift of the binoculus than the other.

Figure III, 1A, shows the sort of record that they sometimes obtain. In the author's opinion, this difference in the slope of the two halves of the graph is the first real demonstration of the existence of a dominant eye in true binocular vision.

Verhoeff (135) has described how darkening one uniocular image, when viewing a pair of cards in a stereoscope, can alter the form of the resulting binocular image. E. F. Fincham has shown me a more interesting form of this experiment. An ordinary circle and dot stereopair are fused, so that the dot appears to be in front of or behind the circle. If the illumination to the two figures is now varied the central dot of the binocular image will be seen to move over towards the position of the dot of the brighter uniocular image without there being any accompanying loss of sense of depth. The experiment can easily be made in a synoptophore if suitable slides are made.

We will not discuss Verhoeff's views on this point here as we shall be dealing with his theory of stereopsis at a later stage. The impression that one gets looking at the slides as the illumination is changing is that the geometry of the figure has remained unchanged, but that the whole solid object has been turned slightly. This is exactly the impression that one would expect if the brain constructed a solid concept of the object based solely on the geometry of the two uniocular images and an alteration of brightness to one of them moved the binoculus, the position from which the mind regards the fused image.

The writer had already reported that he had found that fogging one eye could produce the same effect (35). It was because a shifting of the binoculus with variation of the attention value of the uniocular images, whether caused by changes of brightness or clarity, was the only explanation of the phenomenon that he could think of that he devised the dominance experiments that have just been described and secured the result that he had predicted, on the assumption that this description of the phenomenon was also its explanation. It was found that a neutral density filter had that effect of shifting the centre of projection towards the eye with the brighter image and also that fogging one eye did the same thing. In the stereoscopic form of the experiment the subject's sensation is that the form of the object has been changed, but on the beads seen in the open one's impression on putting up the neutral filter is that one has accidentally moved out of alignment and that one must move back.

In addition to neutral filters and fogging lenses, prisms and size lenses were tried, but no such effect was recorded from either so long as they were not so powerful as to destroy fusion. Conversely neutral density filters were tried on the space eikonometer to see whether they produced any comparable effect on a real three-dimensional target. No effect comparable with the possible accuracy of measurement was found. The test was not repeated with plus lenses as the issue would have been complicated by the fact that they have a geometrical magnifying effect.

Despite the fact that both can be produced with filters this effect is essentially different from the well known Pulfrich effect of the conical pendulum. The first is a static effect while the latter is dynamic; both filters and fogging lenses will produce the former, while a fogging lens has no tendency to cause a pendulum bob to appear to describe an elliptical path. The most generally accepted explanation of the Pulfrich effect is that the filter retards the arrival of the retinal impulse at the occipital cortex, though the mechanism of this retardation is unknown. Such a retardation would explain the Pulfrich effect on geometrical grounds, though it would not explain the Verhoeff-Fincham effect while this shift of the binoculus is unable to explain the Pulfrich effect. A possible unifying explanation of both phenomena is advanced in the last chapter of the book.

The essential difference between man's binocular vision and monocular vision lies in the appreciation of depth given by stereopsis. Monocular vision also gives a sense of depth and in order to appreciate the phenomenon of stereopsis it is necessary to notice the factors on which this monocular depth perception depends. They have been enumerated many times, the listing quoted here is that of Helmholtz (70), though his order has not been adhered to.

The only function which can give a true monocular sensation of difference of distance in which experience plays no part is accommodation. Many attempts have been made to assess its sensitivity, but the writer still knows of no reliable figures. Wundt gave figures of approximately 12 cm. at 250 and 5 cm. at 50 cm. Hillebrand later and with more refined methods came to the conclusion that the sensitivity was lower.

Helmholtz considered that the sense of depth from the parallax of motion ought to be included as a true sensation rather than as a clue dependent on previous experience. The writer's experience from experiments with monocular occlusion convinces him that the trick of moving the head to obtain the successive different perspective views is not innate but acquired. However, this does not prove that the ability to assess the meaning of the change of perspective is not innate. The suggestion is interesting in that it seems to imply that successive images from one eye can make use of the depth perceiving mechanism that is provided for the comparison of the simultaneous images from two eyes. It is unthinkable that any specialized neural mechanism should exist which could be of use only in the event of one eye being lost.

Since it is difficult to see how the same neural mechanism can be used both to compare simultaneous patterns arriving through separate channels and successive patterns arriving by the same channel, the writer is strongly of the opinion that depth appreciation from parallax of motion is solely the result of learning from past experience. Helmholtz divorced it from the " experience " group on the grounds that advantage could not be taken of it in painting a picture, the coming of the movies has shown how effectively it may be used to give solidity to a scene in a " trucking shot " or a " zoom ".

The group that Helmholtz gives as learned by experience are:—

1. Judgment of distance from the size of the retinal image of objects whose approximate size is known, such as men and cattle.

2. The apparent converging of parallel lines in perspective as they recede.

3. The overlapping of one contour by another when a more distant object is partially concealed by another.

4. Clues given by shadows.

5. Aerial perspective or the softening of outline and colour changes of distant objects due to the atmosphere.

Distance judgment from size is too familiar to call for consideration here; it is extensively used in every army for the rapid estimation of the range to targets, and its survey equivalent, the tacheometric theodolite, will be familiar to many readers. Its chief interest to us lies in the fact that we do not have the sensation that objects look smaller as they recede from us. We will return to this point in a later chapter when we consider Luneburg's work.

There used to be a most striking illustration of the importance of perspective to our sense of depth in the Deutsches Museum in Munich. If one stood at a marked spot and looked upwards, with one eye closed, one saw above one a circular gallery with a balustrade carried on slender columns and surmounted by a dome. To anyone with good binocular vision the whole thing collapsed when one opened a second eye, and the fact that it was a painting done on the ceiling became obvious. Yet, so long as one viewed it monocularly and from the correct spot, it was almost impossible to doubt that it was real. Naturally, it had to be viewed from the right place and any movement from that place produced distortions which led to the collapse of the illusion.

In order to illustrate the power of perspective to convey a sense of depth in monocular vision, Miss Georguli has made the writer the drawing reproduced as Figure III, 2. At the writer's request, she has deliberately made the minimum use of all other techniques for portraying depth such as the thinning of lines as they recede, which is the black and white equivalent

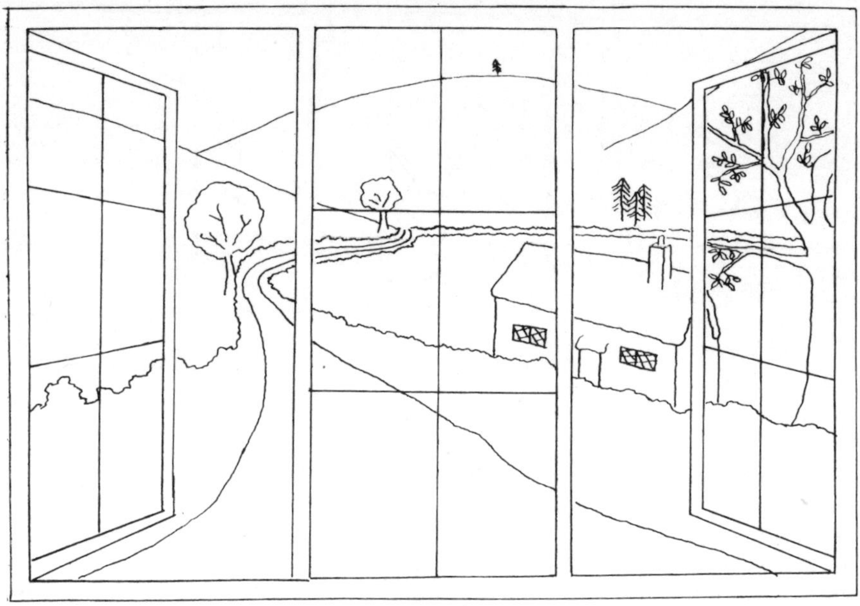

Fig. III. 2.

of aerial perspective. The purpose of the drawing is to show what a much greater sense of depth one obtains if it is viewed with one eye covered. When viewed with two eyes, stereopsis is all the while insisting that the lines are all in the plane of the paper; with stereopsis eliminated perspective is allowed its full weight.

The effect that Miss Georguli has shown can be seen in an even more striking form in those restaurants which have dummy windows with painted street scenes behind them. It is also very noticeable how much more real and solid scenes appear at the cinema to monocular vision than to binocular vision, especially from the seats nearest to the screen.

The discussion of perspective leads us naturally to consider the ambiguities arising from inadequate representation. The best known of these figures is Schroeder's staircase which is typical of the many ambiguous figures which have been designed. It is important to note that the staircase is not drawn in perspective but in isometric projection. If it is drawn in perspective, while it is still possible for those who have practised on the original staircase to invert it, the tendency to do so has largely disappeared for people seeing it for the first time. In the same way careful shading will tend to stabilize it while the addition of a few extra lines of " context " will make it almost impossible to invert it from the staircase to the overhanging feature. These points are illustrated by Figures III, 3, 4 and 5.

Most of us are familiar with the difficulty of seeing a landscape or street scene in pseudoscopic vision when the two pictures of a stereoscopic pair have been interchanged, and it is most entertaining to observe how

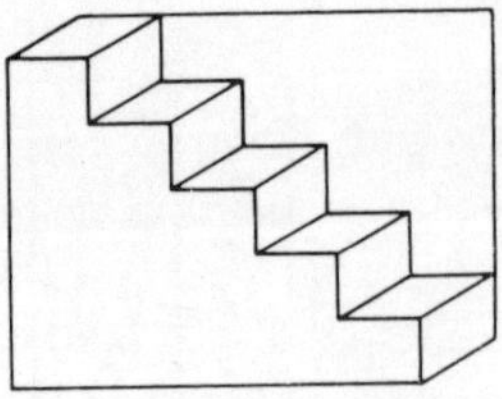

FIG. III 3

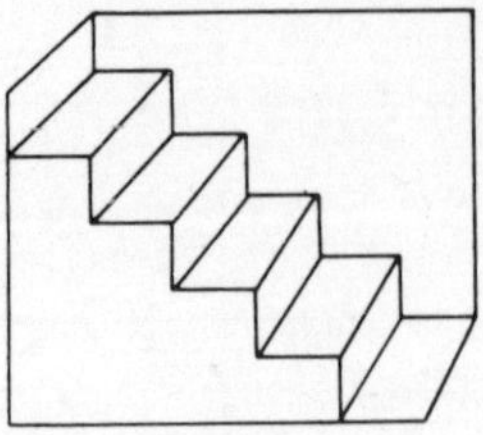

FIG. III 4

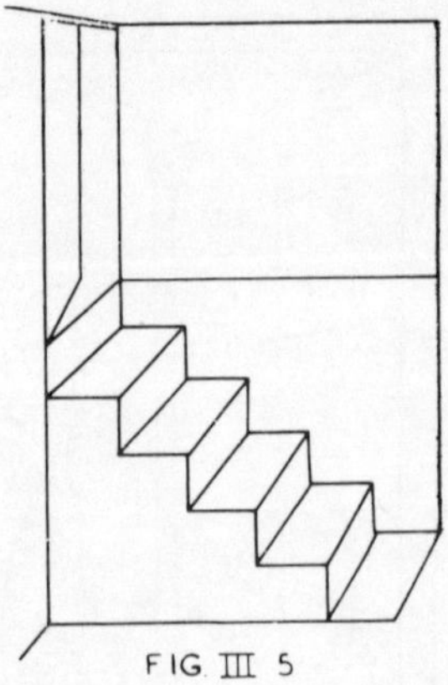

FIG. III 5

much easier it is to obtain pseudoscopy when experience has been embarrassed by turning the picture upside down. Once when adjusting a a pseudoscopic microscope the writer used a cigarette end with a flake of tobacco adhering to it as a test object. Naturally the flake of tobacco passed through the paper and he was pleased to notice a hole for it to pass through. A few days later he showed the hole to a gathering of twenty or thirty opticians, but there was no hole. Cheshire (37) told him that, once, when experimenting with a pair of pseudoscopic binoculars, he noticed that a lamp post across the road appeared to be inside the house opposite and that he could clearly see the hole in the wall through which it must have passed.

These phenomena are interesting because they illustrate the great extent to which past experience and association can influence vision. That they can have no effect on the retinal image is obvious, but there is no question that they do influence what we see.

One of the most convincing demonstrations of the rôle that previous experience plays in vision is the stereoscopic range finder. This instrument is a binocular telescope of moderate magnification with a separation, generally of ten to fifteen feet between its objectives, so as to give the observer an effective interpupillary distance of the object glass separation multiplied by the magnification. In the eyepieces are a stereopair of graticules which are seen in relief in the plane of the image formed by the objectives, and in one telescope tube there is a variable prism system, or its equivalent. Optically the effect of operating the variable prism is to cause the distant scene to approach or recede; it cannot affect the image of the graticule, yet every observer sees the graticules move while the target stays put.

If one trains one of these instruments on a distant hillside and operates its prism, so long as the indicated range is less than that to the solid hillside one can watch the graticule move to and fro across the intervening valley; the moment it reaches the hillside this movement stops. It seems almost as if a flight of birds in formation had crossed the valley and alighted on the hillside, and even though one continues to operate the range-knob the graticule and the hillside appear to be at the same distance until the disparity between the two uniocular images becomes too great to be ignored. When this happens either the graticule dots " burrow " suddenly into the hillside showing holes where they have penetrated or, more usually, the observer breaks fusion on them and they are seen in physiological diplopia instead of stereopsis; they are no longer at any definite distance.

It is clear from the above that convergence is playing no part in assisting the observer to tell whether the target or the graticule is the nearer, since the information that it can supply, namely, that it is the target and not the graticule that is moving, is completely ignored and as soon as one or the other is seen in physiological diplopia one ceases to be able to say which is the nearer except by deductions from past experience, since the graticule, once fusion is lost, is at any distance or no distance from the observer.

Despite the fact that convergence clearly plays no part in stereoscopic range taking, and that, under these circumstances, physiological diplopia leads to complete collapse of one's sense of depth, it is common knowledge that physiological diplopia and a sense of depth are by no means incompatible. Sitting writing in the garden, one can see the path before one, the corner of a writing pad and one's poised pen all approximately in line, but only one of them can be seen singly at a time, yet one is convinced that one can see which is nearer and judge approximately how much nearer.

A little introspection has convinced the author that he sees only one of them at a time as a solid object, and that he makes an estimate of the distance to it, an estimate of an absolute distance capable of being stated in familiar units. While looking at the writing pad it is monocular clues, such as the fact that it is partly obscured by the pen, while it in turn conceals part of the garden path, which show that it is at some distance intermediate between the two, one estimates its distance and compares that estimate with the estimates made of the distance to the pen and to the path.

These estimates of absolute distances clearly cannot be based on disparities between the two uniocular images. Such disparities can give relative differences of distance but always, mathematically, have an infinite number of solutions. There is only one function that can give an absolute value for the distance of an object to an observer, and that is the mind's knowledge of the extent to which the eyes have converged in order to fixate it binocularly.

At first sight it may seem that we have a flat contradiction here. We have just seen that our knowledge of the degree of convergence that we are exercising is unable to tell us that it is the distant scene and not the graticule that moves when we are using a stereoscopic range finder, yet we have also been forced to the conclusion that our knowledge of our convergence is what tells us how far away everyday objects are. This contradiction can easily be resolved by noticing how inexact our appreciation of distance is. Holding a finger in front of one's face at about 18 inches from one's nose, one has no idea whether 17 inches or 19 inches would be the better guess but be confident that the measured distance from one's eyes lies between 16 and 20 inches.

We find, then, that the information of the distance of an object that we can obtain from our knowledge of our convergence has a sensitivity which must be measured in minutes of parallax if not in degrees, whereas the minimum standard for a range taker in the Army or Navy is 12 seconds of parallax and a highly trained observer can observe differences of as little as three seconds of parallax reliably, but it is a difference he is estimating. When he uses convergence to estimate a difference, it seems to the author that he is comparing one estimate with his recollection of another. He has repeatedly observed that if he holds the nib of a pen just far enough from the paper to produce physiological diplopia and then closes one eye after making the most careful estimate that he can of its distance from the paper, he is surprised by the movement necessary to bring the point into contact with the paper.

The writer is well aware of the danger of basing any theory on evidence from introspection, particularly the trained introspection of the experimenter, so closely allied to wishful thinking, so he hopes to support these observations with proper experimental evidence in a later section. Accepting them for the moment, we are forced to conclude that there are two distinct phases to stereoscopic vision. The first is based on our knowledge of the degree of convergence that we are exercising; it gives an actual value for the distance of each object fixated from the observer but only with a very moderate degree of accuracy. The second gives us a difference in distance of two objects in terms of their actual distance from us. This it can do with quite astonishing sensitivity, but it gives no clue whatever to the actual distance of the objects, and in order to give a value to the difference in distance it must be supplied with a scale from some other faculty. Its great value to us lies in the fact that the most useful distance judgment that we are called upon to make in the ordinary affairs of life is to observe when the difference in distance of two points has become zero; that is the information that the surgeon needs to guide his knife, the watchmaker his tweezers, or the clerk his pen.

Of these two, the appreciation of convergence is almost certainly the most ancient. It seems clear that such creatures as the Archer Fish (Toxotes) and the chameleon must have some form of binocular distance judgment, as must also those birds of prey which have two extra foveæ disposed so as to give them bifoveal vision despite the lateral position of their eyes. It will be remembered that all these have demonstrable sensory nerve endings in their extraocular muscles and complete crossings at the chiasma even though they may have a considerable binocular field.

It is reasonable to expect that where the extraocular muscles are well provided with sensory nerve endings and where the eyes have an adequately differentiated macular area, proprioception of convergence may attain to a degree of precision that man's appreciation of convergence lacks. The well known skills of these creatures seems to imply that it does.

It is not until we reach the mammals that we find optic nerve fibres decussating in the chiasma, so that impulses from homonymous halves of the binocular fields of each eye are represented in the same cerebral hemisphere and a central comparison between the uniocular images first becomes possible. We also recall that as this scheme becomes elaborated as we ascend the mammalian scale, so the sensory and proprioceptive terminations disappear from the extraocular muscles. It is for this reason that the author has used the phrase proprioception of convergence when speaking of the lower vertebrates and tried to avoid it when speaking of man.

We shall return later to the evidence for admitting the existence in man of a mental mechanism for constructing a solid concept from two disparate uniocular images without necessarily making use of a knowledge of the degree of convergence in use, as we shall need this evidence when we attempt to form some idea of the method of operation of this mechanism. The immediate point of interest is that man appears to have two distinct forms of stereoscopic sense which he can use separately or in combination without any consciousness of their duality. For the moment, we will ignore that phase of stereopsis which is based on retinal disparities and conclude our consideration of the phenomena associated with stereopsis from convergence and with physiological diplopia.

Wright (155) has found that when acuity of depth perception, with the observer changing fixation from one target to another, is plotted against target separation, the observations for a target separation of 15° fit quite well onto the same smooth curve as those for greater and less separations. This seems to prove that, under the conditions of his experiments and for that target separation, appreciation of convergence is the chief factor in our judgment of depth, and that our estimate of the relative distances of two targets is, under those conditions, a process of comparing the convergence needed to fixate them one after the other. When the observer was required to maintain steady fixation on the reference target no significant recording was possible as one target was only seen monocularly as its image fell on the blind spot of the other eye.

If one makes a fine dot on a piece of paper and approaches a sharp pencil towards it while fixating the dot, the point of the pencil is seen in physiological diplopia. Naturally, as the pencil approaches the dot the diplopic images get closer together as the geometry of the problem requires, but at a certain point very near the dot, the images of the pencil point no longer behave in strict conformity with geometry but begin to come together quicker than they should. It is quite easy to find a point where the two images can be seen moving towards each other, perhaps just fusing and then separating again. The observer must be careful to maintain fixation on the dot as the effect can be simulated by transferring fixation from the dot to the pencil point at any distance, only in this event the dot will be seen in physiological diplopia.

This simple experiment demonstrates that there is a limiting value of retinal disparity below which physiological diplopia does not occur and objects are seen singly simultaneously, even though they are at different visual distances. Another way of describing the same thing is to say that each point of one retina does not correspond rigidly with one point of the other but with a limited area of the other, and that the limits of that area are not very clearly defined. These areas are known as Panum's fusional areas, in recognition of his work on the subject (110).

While it is extremely easy to demonstrate the existence of Panum's areas, or of something equivalent to them, their accurate measurement is a far more difficult matter. Davson (47) gives 3 to 4 minutes as their vertical measurement and 5 to 26 minutes as their horizontal. A recent attempt at a determination by the author (31) gave a mean value of 25. It seems certain that their size varies considerably from one individual to the next and that it may be possible to enlarge them by training. If this is so, it is clear that, though they must have an anatomical basis, they have no physical limits and our statement above means no more than that individuals vary in their mental power of reconciling image disparities and achieving true fusion despite them.

This conception tempts us once again to consider the question that we discussed in Chapter I of whether there exists a fusion centre in the brain. We have seen that it is unlikely that there is a separate cerebral structure in any way analogous to a nucleus which is a centre responsible for fusion and nothing else, and, in the writer's view, it is probable that fusion is part of the function of the area striata. This would account adequately for the variability of the function and its trainability. The biggest difficulty that confronts us on this hypothesis is to account for the rare cases where the fusion sense appears to be lacking without any accompanying visual defect.

Worth (154) postulated a fusion centre chiefly in order to be able to assume deficiencies of it in order to account for horror fusionis. The author has seen a number of cases of horror fusionis, but in all but three he has been able to show a good reason for their inability to fuse. Detailed consideration of these is, perhaps, best postponed to the section where we consider the evidence afforded by abnormal conditions.

CHAPTER IV

SOME INVESTIGATIONS OF BINOCULAR VISION

This chapter can scarcely have a better starting point than the classic researches of Sir Charles Sherrington. These stand midway in time between the pioneer work of Helmholtz and his contemporaries and the sophisticated though revolutionary twist that Luneburg has given to our ideas on the subject. Sherrington's work on binocular vision was the logical, subjective sequel of his pioneer work on reflexes which laid the foundations for the modern view of the ocular reflexes which we considered in Chapter II.

Sherrington's method of investigating the mental integration of the two uniocular images (125) was by means of a lantern which presented fuseable patches of light to the two eyes which could be made to flicker at known and controllable rates, and whose relative brightness could also be controlled. In order to ensure that neither target was being suppressed, one had a horizontal line across it while the other had a vertical; so long as both were present in consciousness the subject saw an even circular patch of light with two lines on it forming a cross.

The first effect that he recorded is that while flicker was extinguished at a slightly higher speed if the two eyes were stimulated alternately than if they were stimulated simultaneously, the difference was far too small to suggest any sort of direct summation, which seems to go some way towards killing the oft-repeated suggestion that in binocular vision the two eyes function alternately. Another result was that the rate for extinction of flicker was almost identical whether two eyes were stimulated simultaneously, or one eye alone was stimulated.

If the frequency of the light stimulating one eye was twice that of the light stimulating the other, flicker was extinguished at some intermediate rate, higher than that required by the more rapidly flashing light if it were acting alone on one eye, but substantially below that which the slower light would require under similar circumstances. This effect was observed, with some variation of the critical speed, whether the high speed light was brighter or dimmer than the slow one. This experiment was repeated with half the high speed spot blacked out, so that one eye saw two slow speed spots while the other a low speed spot and half of the high speed spot. The subjective sensation was of two spots equally illuminated.

Sherrington then went on to use his flicker lantern to investigate the summation of brightness by two eyes. The arrangement that he used was such that each eye saw two spots of light which the two eyes saw as three, the centre spot being the result of fusing the top spot seen by one eye with the lower spot seen by the other. It is obviously easy to arrange that the two fused spots should be of the two brightnesses to be summed, while the others can be used as photometer spots. The surprising result that he obtained was that the resulting binocular sensation of brightness was slightly higher than the mean of the two uniocular brightnesses. The following table summarises the results:—

Right eye field brightness	*Left eye field brightness*	*Binocular brightness*
1,000	250	680
1,000	350	750
1,000	550	835
1,000	750	920
1,000	1,000	1,000

Finally Sherrington investigated the difference between binocular fusion and physical fusion resulting from superimposing the two images on the retina of one eye by optical means. The targets that he used were again evenly illuminated light patches, but this time one of them had a broad black bar across it. With the two targets evenly illuminated the bar was present in the single image however formed. When the illumination of the target with the bar was reduced sufficiently the bar disappeared from consciousness. Where the two images were presented optically to a single eye a reduction of illumination of 84 per cent to the target with the bar was necessary to cause it to disappear. If the images were presented to the two eyes and fused by the subject's binocular vision, the necessary reduction of illumination became 96 per cent; naturally, if this target were seen alone, an even greater reduction was necessary.

In his discussion of these experiments, Sherrington says,

> " Our experiments show, therefore, that during binocular regard of an objective image each uniocular mechanism develops independently a sensual image of considerable completeness. The singleness of the binocular perception results from union of these elaborated uniocular sensations. The singleness is therefore the product of a synthesis that works with already elaborated sensations contemporaneously proceeding.
>
> The cerebral seat of right eye and left eye images are thus shown to be separate. Conducting paths no doubt interconnect them, but are shown to be unnecessary for visual unification of the two images. The unification of a sensation of composite source is evidently associated with a neuron arrangement different from that which obtains in the synthesis of a reflex movement by the convergence of allied arcs upon its final common path.
>
> Here we seem to have, therefore, contemporaneity in itself sufficient for sensual synthesis, without necessarily any spatial fusion of the neural processes or mechanisms involved, i.e., without spatial confluence to a unit apparatus."

This is a most remarkable passage, the more so when one remembers that it was written more than forty years ago. Reading it now, however, it is necessary to call attention to certain points where later research has not borne out Sherrington's anticipations. He says that the cerebral seats of the right and left eye images are shown to be separate; his requirements are, however, met by the modern view. All that he has shown is that the two eyes initially stimulate separate cells in the cortex. There is nothing in his experiments, or in a liberal reading of the above quotation, that insists that these cells must be far apart. We know now that they are, in fact, intimately intermingled.

The reason for quoting this statement at length and for presuming to attempt to interpret Sherrington is that that passage is sometimes quoted as authority for the proposition that true fusion does not exist. Even Verhoeff (136) has lent the weight of his reputation to this supposition. Elliman (54) has put this theory most clearly in the form of two " rules ": " That projection is as from the stimulated nerve ending." " That fusion takes place after projection." He illustrates this by comparing binocular vision to binocular hearing, a fallacy that has already been disposed of.

The writer prefers the description which Sherrington gives a page before the paragraph quoted above:

> " The inference is that only after the sensations initiated from right and left 'corresponding points' have been elaborated, and have reached a dignity and definiteness well amenable to introspection, does interference between the two (left and right) eye-systems occur. The binocular sensation attained seems combined from right and left uniocular sensations elaborated independently."

The two passages are quoted verbatim in order to make it clear that while the first-quoted could be used out of its context to support views such as Verhoeff's, the two together make it quite clear that this was not Sherrington's own interpretation of his work.

The other set of classic experiments which have been quoted regularly in support of widely diverging views are those of Langlands (81) on the relationship between duration of illumination and stereoscopic acuity. The results are so well known that it is unnecessary to quote them in detail. Briefly, he found that some slight sense of depth was observed even when the test objects were only visible for a hundredth of a second or less, with little further loss when the period of illumination was reduced still further. As the period of visibility was increased, a sudden change in sensitivity was observed in the neighbourhood of one-tenth of a second, but after one second's exposure the rate of increase was again very slow. In view of the fact that this sudden improvement in stereoacuity occurs at the point where the period of illumination of the test objects is approximately equal to the reaction time of the extraocular muscles, some workers have argued that these experiments support the view that stereopsis is a process of appreciation of the degree of convergence being exercised. It seems to the writer that the observed facts can be explained at least equally well by noting that the reaction time of the extraocular muscles is also the least time needed for accurate binocular fixation.

We have already seen that knowledge of the degree of convergence in use plays an important part in our sense of depth and that it is probably all important in our judgment of short distances, but the question of how great a part it plays in our estimates of small differences of distance is an entirely separate one and one which Langlands' work alone seems quite unable to answer. If our estimate of differences in distance is based on a comparison of the convergence to one target with the convergence to another, one would expect that the steepest point of Langlands' curve would occur at an exposure time of not less than twice the time needed for accurate fixation. At the moment, the author does not know of any adequate estimate of this time, but the flicker and fusion experiments of Winkelman (148) quoted in a previous chapter suggest that this time is longer rather than shorter. Information is also needed on the relationship between the angular distance of the direction of gaze and the target to be fixed and the exposure time necessary to fix it.

The author has lately conducted a brief series of experiments on the factors affecting stereoscopic acuity, expressed in terms of the minimum parallax angle recognised reliably. The targets used were beads of approximately 6 mm. diameter and were invisibly suspended and seen against a black background through a mask which hid all other relevant objects. For the great part of this work he was his own test subject for reasons of convenience, in particular that he trains very readily to a steady optimum which is repeatable with a considerable degree of reliability. As only two beads were used, only two answers were possible, right nearest or left nearest, the setting made by the examiner was determined by using the London Telephone Directory as a book of random sampling numbers, so as to avoid the risk of the subject trying to read the examiner's mind when judgment became difficult. Eight right answers out of ten were accepted as an end point as a preliminary experiment indicated that this was the most sensitive and repeatable criterion. No form of head fixation was used, as at the working distance adopted, 3·4 metres, accidental head movements could only introduce second order effects on subjects capable of a stereoscopic acuity of 5 seconds and better.

Figure IV 1 records the results. A shows the change in stereo-acuity recorded for varying separations of the two beads when the subject was free to change fixation from one to the other. It is interesting to note that there is a suggestion that there seems to be a maximum between the two first points, which is in good agreement with Hirsch and Weymouth (72) finding that stereoscopic acuity is greatest when the separation between two targets is 19 minutes and falls off both above and below this value. B gives the same information for a subject maintaining steady fixation on one of the two beads.

Another method of analysis is to present the second target at different distances before and behind the reference target in a random manner and to plot the percentage of right or wrong answers against the difference in distance between the two targets, as in Figure IV, 2. The maximum steepness of the slope of the curve being a measure of the acuity realised.

Wright and Ellerbrook used methods of this sort while Hirsch and Weymouth and Colenbrander used criteria similar to those used by the author. Both systems have very real advantages but, unfortunately, a direct comparison of the results from the different systems is generally impossible unless there is a substantial overlap.

In the paper referred to in the last chapter (155), Wright gave some preliminary results of an investigation into the stereo-acuity realised when the subject was allowed to change fixation from one target to the

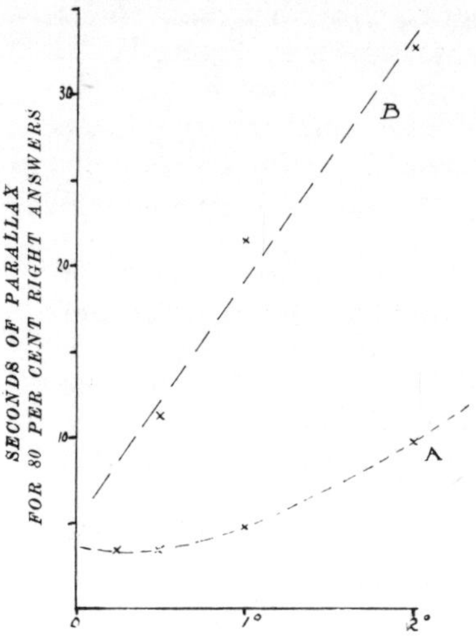

Fig. IV. 1.

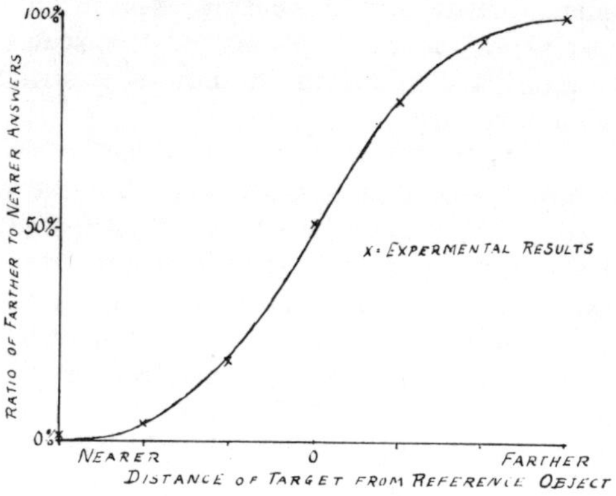

Fig. IV. 2.

other and when he was required to maintain fixation on the reference target. Although this work is still in progress, the author has had the opportunity, through the courtesy of Dr. Wright, to see the results so far obtained and to try to correlate them with his own. Unfortunately, the only result is to make it clear that he must greatly extend the range of his own observations before such an attempt can serve any useful purpose.

Colenbrander (39) has found that if the visual acuity of an observer's eyes is reduced with plus lenses, the reduction in his stereoacuity is directly proportional to the amount of the blurring, while for monocular blurring

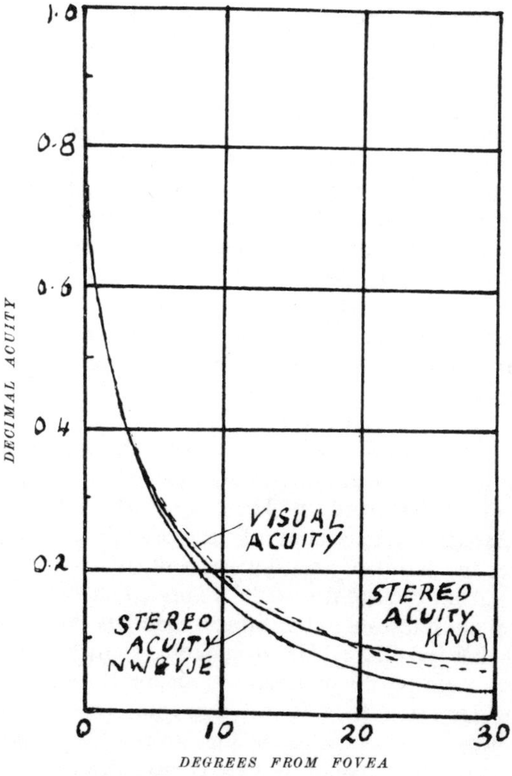

Fig. IV. 3.
(from *Amer. Jl. Optom.*, Dec., 1949)

the fall is proportional to the square root of the blurring. It is interesting to compare these findings with those shown in Figure IV, 3, which gives some results published by Ellerbrook (53) which correlate stereo-acuity for increasing separations with the visual acuity of the peripheral retina. Naturally, the scales adopted are arbitrary but the similarity in shape of the curves is striking and supports the findings of Colenbrander.

In connection with the effect of visual acuity on stereo-acuity, it seems reasonable to deal here with the results obtained by Schäffer and Erner. These workers have reported (122) that they have recorded an improvement in stereoscopic acuity from placing a filter in front of one eye. As their experiments were conducted on a small scale, it is impossible to apply any form of statistical analysis to their published results. One fact stands out clearly in their report and must be accepted; that is that placing a coloured filter in front of one eye resulted in an improvement in the stereoscopic acuity of two observers considerably greater than the precision of measurement that they claimed. This result has worried the writer considerably as he could not, at first, see any explanation for it. He accordingly endeavoured to repeat their experiments, firstly using the space eikonometer as a stereo-acuity meter (35), and secondly on his standard stereo-acuity set up. In each case he was the subject of the experiment, and in neither case was it possible for him to know the result before the experiment was complete. In each case, every filter tried, whether coloured or neutral, lowered his stereoscopic acuity. It was therefore necessary to search for some factor that could explain these contradictory results, and to hope that it would be one which would furnish a more plausible explanation of the Schäffer and Erner results than they, themselves, or any other workers have so far offered. It seemed likely that the reconciling factor would prove to be some idiosyncrasy of his own visual equipment. Naturally, the writer's own vision has been experimented on very extensively and he is well acquainted with the characteristics of his eyes. Beyond a small amount of myopia and a trace of astigmatism, he believes them to be as near perfect as one dare hope, certainly his corrected acuity of 6/3 leaves little to be desired. He therefore started to search for some unsuspected excellence and found, as he has recorded in an earlier chapter, that he has an unusually small chromatic difference of magnification with the result that, far from being able to improve on his acuity, any prism introduced monocularly for this purpose in the manner described by Hartridge (67) reduces it. He therefore suggests that the improvement of stereo-acuity recorded by Schäffer and Erner was the result of an improvement in visual acuity from the filter acting as a partial monochromator. This effect has been claimed by certain commercial interests in the States. He has taken no steps to pursue the matter further as this explanation seems convincing to him, and the point does not seem to be of great importance. This explanation is supported by the fact that they found a greater improvement for some colours than others.

A phenomenon which is not strictly one of binocular vision, since it only occurs under artificial conditions, is retinal rivalry. When the two eyes are presented with images which cannot be fused, they tend to alternate in consciousness. The patterns most commonly used to illustrate the effect are two squares, one shaded with diagonal lines running down from left to right, and the other from right to left. When these two are combined in a stereoscope, the result is not a chequer board, nor is it a field uniformly shaded one way or the other. The result is a square completely covered with diagonal lines some running one way and some another, but none of which cross one another. The field is filled with portions selected, apparently at random, from the two uniocular fields, nor is this field stable, on the contrary it is in a continuous state of flux, now one set of diagonals predominating and now the other.

The interest of the phenomenon lies in the fact that it gives us a useful tool for investigating binocular vision. For instance, it has been suggested that the respective times during which each uniocular pattern predominated in the binocular field might be a guide as to which should be considered the master eye. Similarly the presence of retinal rivalry at the junction of two fusible but dissimilar patterns, such as the letters F and L fused to form an E, is far more conclusive proof that there is no suppression than if the letter E is seen quite solidly.

Davson (47) states as a general law that when dissimilar patterns are presented to the two eyes, the predominant field along an edge will be that in which the edge lies. He illustrates this by the case of two bars, one vertical and the other horizontal, each presented to one eye so as to form a cross. Where the two bars cross each has two edges crossing the solid block of the other, along these edges the eye that sees them is dominant, so the observer sees a cross with a clear black square in the middle with a white surround, clean cut at the edge next to the square but fading into the solid bar of the cross as the dominance passes from one eye to the other.

Bárány (11) has reported that when, during retinal rivalry, one or other eye suppresses, the pupil of that eye fails to respond to light stimuli. This suggests that suppression, at any rate under conditions of retinal rivalry, is an inhibition that extends to sub-cortical levels, and that the inhibition extends to the retina via the centrifugal fibres of the optic nerves. Bárány and Halldén (12) have also shown that the rate of alternation of dominance between the two eyes can be profoundly affected by drugs, which act on the central nervous system, such as amytal, chloral and ethyl alcohol. They have reported promising results from the use of alcohol in the treatment of one case of amblyopia in squint.

An interesting use of the retention in consciousness of an edge or end is the placing of marker gaps in lines of stereoscopic figures to ensure that the line has not been suppressed by the eye to which it has been presented. The gap having edges makes the field in which it occurs dominant in its immediate neighbourhood, and so is always present in the conscious image. Verhoeff (136) made use of these gaps in the figures which he used to illustrate his theory of binocular vision. We shall make even more free use of them in discussing his theory.

Verhoeff considers that binocular lustre, or stereoscopic lustre, is a limiting case of retinal rivalry where the alternation is between individual units of the retina rather than between individual elements of the uniocular fields. The effect is shown very well by the stereopair, Fig. IV, 4, copied from Helmholtz's " Physiological Optics ". When they are fused the percept is a lustrous crystal rather like graphite. It will be noticed that the lustre extends onto the ground and is not confined to the parts of the figure seen in stereoscopic relief. It is for this reason that I prefer the name binocular lustre to the older term. Dove, who first observed the effect, considered that it was due to the different stimulation of the two eyes simulating the explanation which he advanced for metallic lustre, namely that the true surface of the metallic object reflected white light and that the coloured light reflected by the superficial layers of the object was seen through this white light.

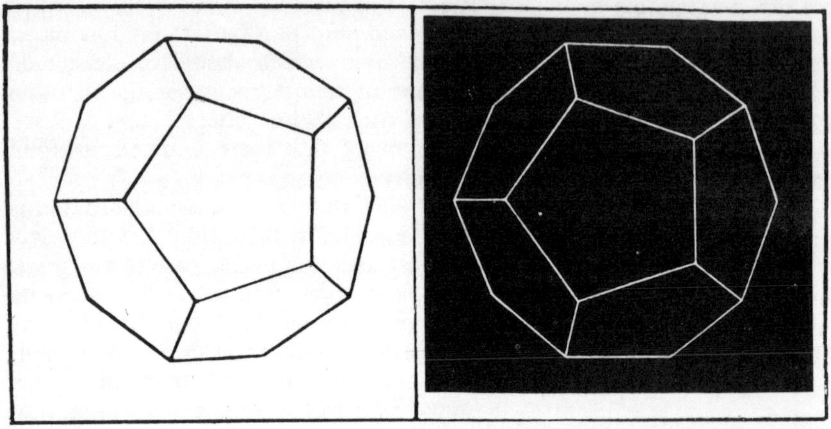

Fig. IV. 4.

Helmholtz rejected this theory and held that metallic lustre was due to the object reflecting more light into one eye than the other, and that the contrasting visual fields simulated this effect. He pointed out that a lustrous body surrounded by coloured objects will often reflect light of different colours into the two eyes. Against this view is the fact that metallic lustre is seen monocularly. It seems to the writer that the true explanation of metallic lustre is that the micro structure of the surface is such that while the whole surface appears flat and may even give a low grade specular reflection, a considerable aggregate area is made up of facets of the order of the wave length of light behaving as reflecting gratings and adjoining retinal elements are differently illuminated. The result is that corresponding points in the two eyes will almost all be receiving light differing in intensity and/or colour. When the eyes are presented with fusible patterns differing in colour, e.g. one black and one white, the impression conveyed to the conscious cells is essentially the same as if the contrasting stimuli were divided between the two eyes, as the mind has no means of telling which eye supplied which element of the percept, and makes the fullest possible use of information supplied to it.

We need not discuss corresponding points at length here, as they come more naturally into the next chapter in connection with the consideration of abnormal retinal correspondence. Here it is enough to note that to think of corresponding points as such is too rigid and narrow a simile for what must occur. When two objects at different apparent distances are seen, the images of both objects cannot fall on corresponding points of the two retinæ, and we are forced to realize that these corresponding points are more properly pictured as corresponding areas within which points may correspond with each other. Many efforts have been made to estimate their size, but I do not know of any reliable measurements. Davson quotes from 5 to 26 minutes for the horizontal measurement, and 3 to 4 for the vertical. It seems probable that they can be enlarged by training and also that they vary in size in different parts of the visual field.

The author has found (29) that the retinal disparity between targets which is compatible with single binocular vision varies greatly with the nature of the targets and their separation. Two vertical black threads in the median plane could not both be seen singly against a white background when their distances were 300 cm. and 315 cm. from the observer. Two white beads at 300 cm. and 330 cm. could be seen without diplopia so long as their vertical separation was not less than about 15 minutes of arc, whereas when the farther bead was moved back to 400 cm. the vertical separation necessary increased to about $1\frac{1}{2}^{\circ}$. These figures varied appreciably for different observers, but the form of the relationship was reasonably constant. A similar relationship was found to hold for horizontal separation.

It is not surprising that it should be impossible to see the two threads in line even for such small disparities as 4 minutes, since in order to do so the mind would have to suppress both disparate images and assume that an object that both eyes could see was hidden by a nearer one. The writer is indebted to Murroughs and Cristakos (106) for the criticism which brought out this point.

Certain anomalies of correspondence have been recorded in normal eyes and were the subject of an enormous amount of experimental work during the latter half of the last century. Helmholtz gives Volkmann (140) the credit for having started this work. It was extended and amplified by many other workers including himself, Dastich, and Hering. Starting with the two points of fixation as corresponding points, the second proposition is that the two retinal horizons correspond. It was here that the first anomaly was recorded when Volkmann found that the monocular retinal horizon dipped down on the side of the eye in use. The angle recorded varied considerably between individuals and in some cases it varied with the state of rest of convergence, but the sign of the deviation was always the same, and the average value of about half a degree was fully four times the statistical probable error of the experiments. These workers also found that the apparent vertical meridians of the two eyes, separately, diverge upwards to an even greater extent than the horizontals dip outwards, the average included angle being of the order of two degrees; the average error deduced for these experiments was somewhat larger than for the horizon series, but smaller in comparison with the recorded deviations.

The next proposition about corresponding points that they investigated was that points on the apparent vertical meridians equidistant from the point of fixation are corresponding points; here no anomaly was found. Volkmann failed to demonstrate any incongruity along the horizontal, but later experiments show that Kundt's illusion (79) is almost universal. Practically everyone who tries to bisect a line using the right eye only, makes the right half too big and makes the contrary error when using the left eye only.

With the modern mathematical descriptive approach to such problems, the compiling of such measurements loses much of its significance and their interest becomes largely historical, but it is still interesting to read that von Kries, in his notes to the third edition of Helmholtz's "Physiological Optics," regards Kundt's illusion as the final confirmation of the Hering-Hillebrand horopter deviation. With the descriptive viewpoint speculations such as Hering's, that the subjective distance between points was a function not of the arc but of the chord on the retina, lose all interest.

The nineteenth century was the time when the scientist was in the habit of saying that he could not understand anything unless he could make a model of it. Perhaps the author may be forgiven for saying that this attitude seems to him to survive in many schools of psychology long after the physicist has outgrown it. During the second half of the century a great deal of work was spent on endeavouring to determine the form of the horopter, and one feels that much of it must have been designed to identify it with Müller's circle, the circle passing through the two eyes and the point of fixation which is the geometrical locus of points of equal subtense angle.

Studies on the form of the horopter were continued into the later twenties of this century and for our purposes it is sufficient to record the form generally accepted now. Duke-Elder (49a) gives the nearer ones as curves concave towards the observer approximating to a straight line at a distance of about two metres, beyond which distance the central portion of the curve is convex towards the observer. Among the latest and most meticulous studies have been those made at the Dartmouth Eye Institute under Ames (108). Fig. IV, 5, illustrates their findings.

Horopter experiments are very well known; experiments on lines more or less at right angles to the horopters are far less well known. Hillebrand is usually credited with being the first to conduct "alley" experiments. Perhaps Blumenfeld's repeat work (19) shows the point which seems important now most clearly. A subject is seated facing a series of pairs of vertical wires, one of each pair on each side of his median plane, each pair farther from him by a constant interval than the previous pair, and the separation of each pair under his control except for the farthest pair, which are fixed equidistant from the median plane. The subject is required to arrange the remaining pairs so that each shall be the same distance from the median plane as the fixed wires. He arranges them in a characteristic curve very consistently.

If the instructions to the subject are now varied and he is asked to arrange the wires in two parallel straight lines passing through the two fixed wires equidistant from the median plane, he again places them in a characteristic curve which, again, is consistently repeated, but which is not the same curve as that in which he places them when the emphasis is on keeping the separation between the individual pairs of wires constant.

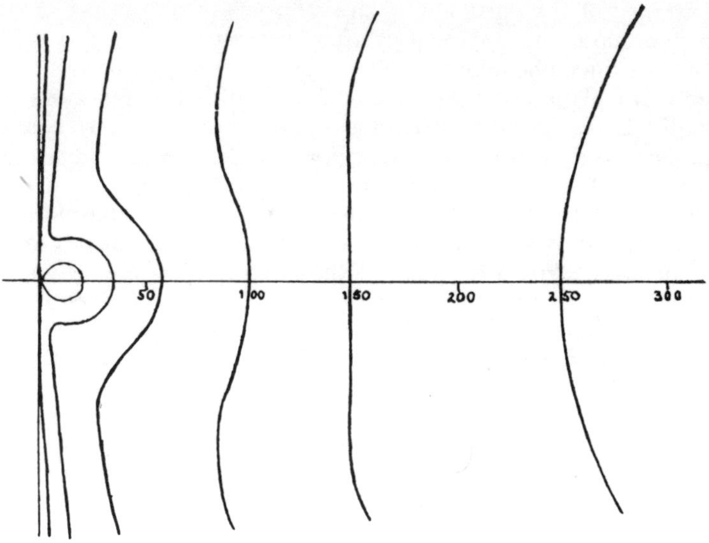

Fig. IV. 5.

The difference between the curves resulting from the instruction to keep the separation of the walls of the alley constant and the instruction to keep them parallel is greater than the random variation on either instruction and is quite consistent. Yet in Euclidean geometry the two instructions are synonymous.

Consideration of this apparent contradiction taken with the form of the horopter led Ames to construct three open-ended " rooms " of three sides, a floor and a ceiling, which proved indistinguishable to binocular vision. One was " honest ", being a true parallelepiped with truly rectangular window patterns painted on its walls, one with concave walls and suitably distorted windows was smaller, while another with convex walls and the appropriate window was larger. Yet, not only to monocular vision but to binocular vision, these three rooms were indistinguishable, they were congruent.

Another phenomenon, which belongs as much to monocular vision as to binocular vision, deserves to be considered alongside those which we have been describing; that is the constancy of our sensation or impression of the size of an object, irrespective of its distance from us. We have already noticed that the apparent size or angular subtense of familiar objects can be used as an aid to estimating distance, but this is a process of conscious introspection and our starting point is our estimate of the size of the distant object and not its angular subtense. The important point is that we do not mistake a child four hundred yards away for a man six hundred yards away, even though its angular subtense is the same as the man's. This fact is, if we think about it, most surprising but it is so familiar that generations of writers have passed it by. There appears to be some evidence that the power is not innate, yet early in life the sun is seen as far larger than an orange ten yards away. This phenomenon of the constancy of the sensation of size irrespective of distance is contrary to our expectations based on Euclidean geometry.

The last three phenomena, the horopter, the alleys, and size constancy are the main planks of Luneburg's analysis of binocular vision, but as this chapter is a review of the experimental evidence that has to be accounted for, Luneburg's mathematical description will be held for the last chapter.

We have already touched on the use that can be made of stereograms as a means of investigating binocular vision. Their convenience as a means of presenting separate targets with controlled disparities to the two eyes is obvious. Fig. IV, 6, shows the simplest possible stereogram; it consists of only four dots, two seen by each eye, and it gives a sensation of depth. The elimination of any one of those dots destroys all sensation of depth. It is reproduced as a demonstration that suppression cannot play an essential part in stereopsis. It is important to note that the two dots resulting from fusing the two pairs are vertically above each other. Fig. IV, 7, shows the same stereogram, but with one dot transferred from the left eye to the right to show how clearly diplopia would be seen were it present, while Fig. IV, 8, is Fig. IV, 6, with the disparity increased to the point where fusion of both pairs at once is difficult. If the lower dots are fused the upper two may be seen *both* trying to move towards a central position; some observers can avoid diplopia on the two resulting dots, others cannot.

Fig. IV, 9, is an attempt to illustrate an effect described by Verhoeff (135). If two circles each with a diameter slightly inclined as in this figure are fused, the resulting line is seen in the median plane. If, now, a neutral filter is introduced before one eye so as to dim down half of one of the two images as indicated in the figure, the resultant line will be seen to be bent towards the component in the bright field. Fig. IV, 10, shows what is seen, the marker gap shows that the dimmer component has not been eliminated but is still contributing to the resultant. These stereograms do not show the effect nearly as well as the original experiment but it is sometimes observable and they seem the only way to attempt to reproduce it on paper. The object of trying to show it is to illustrate the fact that a straight line in a monocular component does not necessarily make a straight line in the binocular resultant.

Fig. IV, 11, is a modification of another stereogram of Verhoeff's (136). In the original there is no marker gap in the portion of the upright line which lies inside the right hand circle. Verhoeff claims that this portion has disappeared from consciousness and has been replaced by the white space in the other uniocular image. The addition of a marker gap shows that it has been fused with one or other of the two parallel lines in the left hand image. The gap may be seen on either of them almost at will and the writer has occasionally seen the central portion of the right hand upright with its gap pass from one line of the binocular picture to the other. Whichever line it fuses with stands out in relief, the left hand one in front of the circle and the right hand one behind.

Fig. IV, 12, is a simplification of another of Verhoeff's stereograms from the same paper. There appears to be at least three ways of seeing it. Verhoeff saw the whole of the arrow in stereoscopic relief despite the fact that he always saw the marker gap on the radius. The author

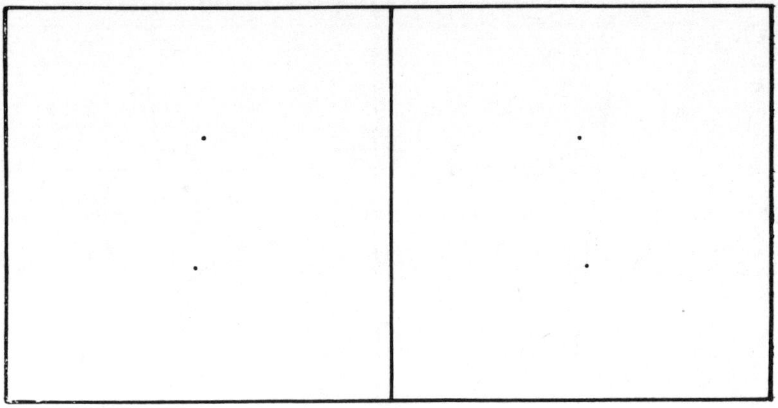

FIG. IV 6.

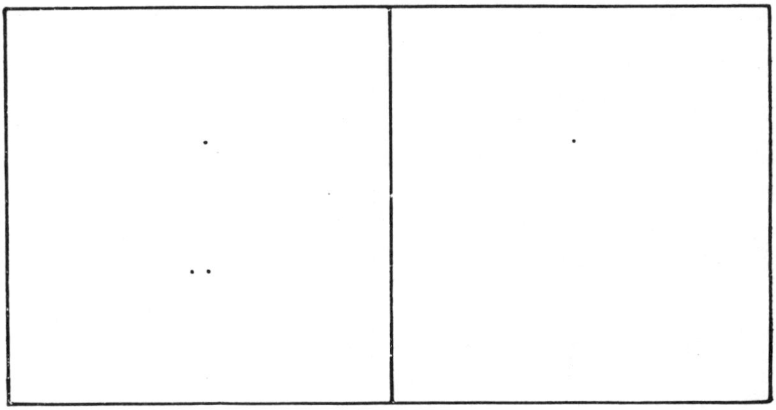

FIG. IV 7.

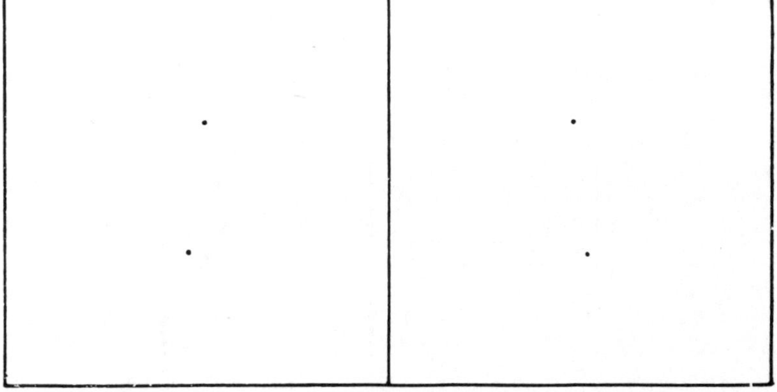

FIG. IV 8.

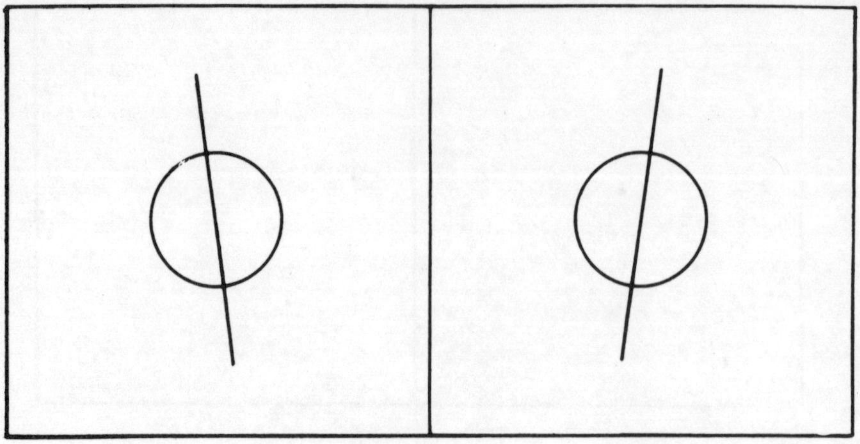

FIG. IV 9.

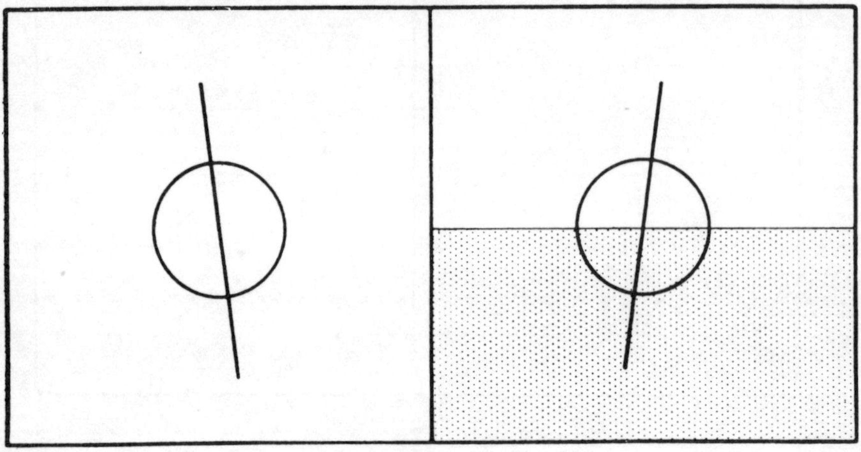

FIG. IV 10.

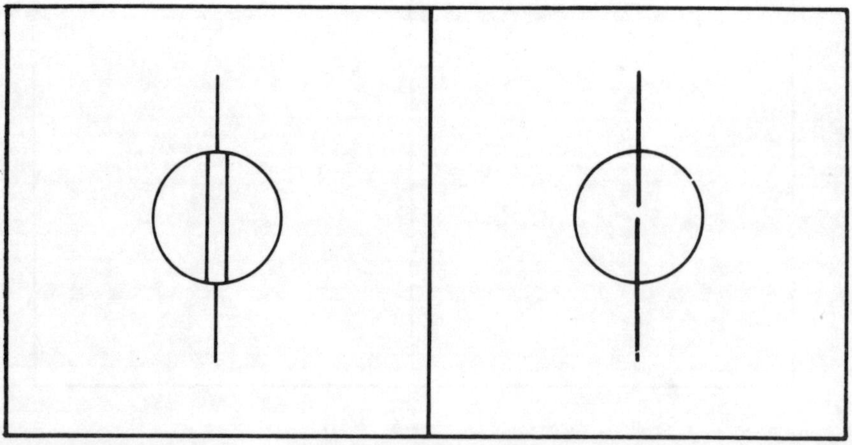

FIG. IV 11.

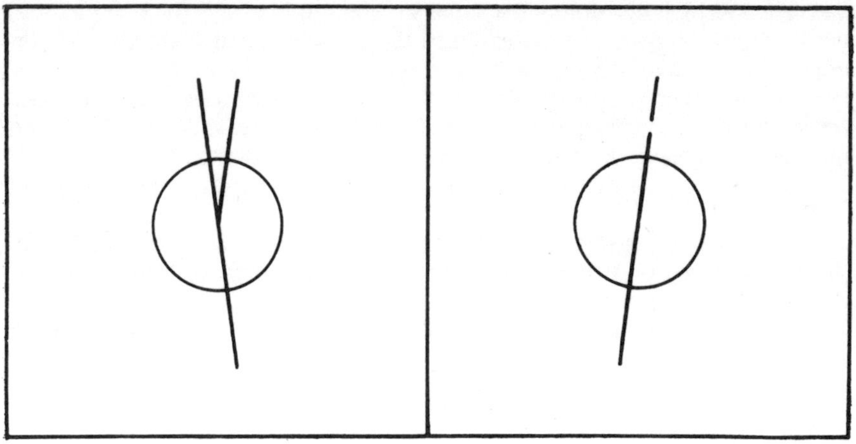

FIG. IV 12.

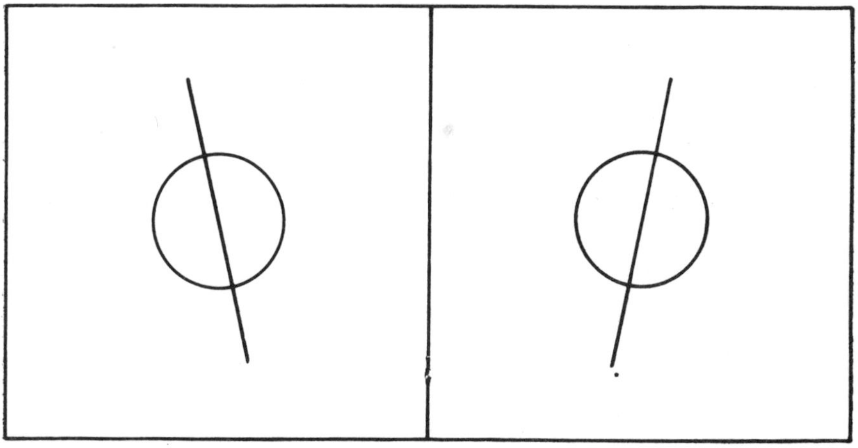

FIG. IV 13.

sees it either with the top half of the arrow in stereoscopic relief and its tail bent into the plane of the circle to form a second radius symmetrical with that in the left eye component, or he sees it as Verhoeff describes it with the whole arrow in relief in the median plane and the marker gap on the arrow not on the radius. Boeder (20) very tactfully sees it either as Verhoeff does or in the second of the author's two ways, but when he tried it he did not see the arrow tail in the plane of the circle. The importance of this figure lies in the way in which it illustrates one's power to see what one wants. It was designed by a first class observer to illustrate his theory of binocular vision, and he saw what he wanted. The writer believes himself to be a very good observer but he does not accept Verhoeff's theory. His own views required that he should see something different, so he saw what his theory demanded. Boeder showed himself to be a man of great tact and charm, as always.

Fig. IV, 13, is essentially the same stereogram but with the extra radius omitted and the disparity increased to the point where it is difficult, if not impossible, to avoid diplopia on the whole of the arrow at once. It is included in order to illustrate the way in which the two uniocular images curve towards, or away from the median fused portion as the disparity reduces or increases as one looks from one part of the arrow to another. This may indicate a mechanism whereby a sense of depth can be achieved without fusion.

The other method by which the uniocular image may be modified in shape is the use of size lenses. These are lenses of zero dioptric power which none the less have a small magnifying power. Fig. IV, 14, shows such a lens. Essentially it consists of a positive surface separated from

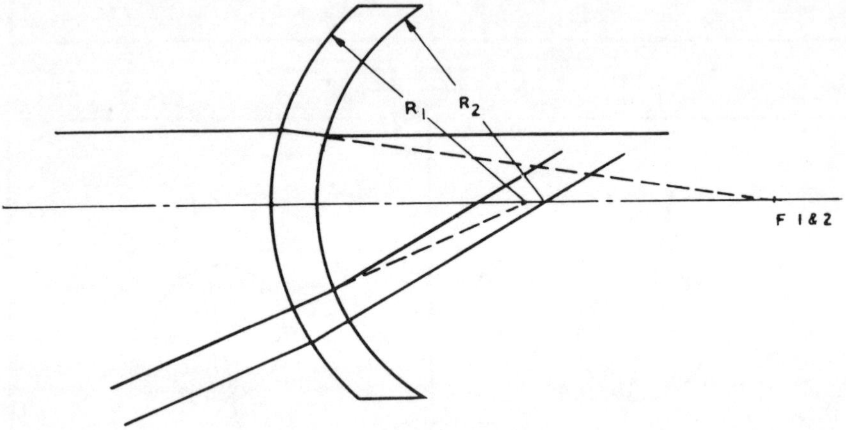

FIG. IV 14.

the negative surface which exactly neutralises it. This is, in effect, the simple Galilean telescope of the elementary textbook, the only difference being that it is made from one piece of glass or plastic. If a beam of parallel light falls on it it will emerge parallel, but unless it is an axial beam the angle that it makes with the axis will have changed. The ratio of the sign of the angle made with the axis by the emergent beam to that of the entering beam is the magnification. A lens 5 mm. thick with a front surface of $+$ 6·00 D, and a rear surface of $-$ 6·12 D, would have a magnifying power of 1·02 or 2 per cent. As some erroneous diagrams of these lenses have been published, Fig. IV, 14, shows the condition for neutralization, namely that the foci of the two surfaces should coincide, and traces a few rays through. Note that the centres of curvature of the two surfaces are separated by approximately half the thickness of the glass, so that a ray normal to the first surface will not be normal to the second, and so will be refracted away from the normal on passing from a denser to a less dense medium. A ray is shown directed at the centre of curvature of the first surface and a ray passing through the centre of curvature of the second surface; it will be seen that they enter and leave the lens parallel to each other. The thickness of the lens has been exaggerated for the sake of clarity. A ray parallel to the axis is also shown; it is still parallel to it when it emerges.

If such a lens is made from cylindrical surfaces, with their axes parallel, instead of spherical surfaces, it will still be a Galilean telescope, but in one meridian only, the other meridian being plane parallel. Such a lens magnifies in one direction only so that a circle seen through it will be distorted into an ellipse with its major axis at right angles to the axis of the lens. Lines crossing at right angles will suffer the scissors distortion shown by cylindrical lenses with a dioptric power, unless, just as with the astigmatic lens, they lie in the planes of the principal meridians of the lens.

With such lenses it is easy to make small alterations to individual uniocular images which are almost inappreciable to monocular vision, but which suffice to disorientate binocular vision intensely. Generally speaking, the results are such as would be expected from geometrical considerations. ·A meridional size lens with its axis vertical placed before the right eye causes objects on the right of the field of vision to appear farther off, and objects which are on the left to seem nearer, the ground seems to slope downhill to the right. A pair of them, one before each eye, with their axes inclining towards each other upwards cause things to slope down away from you, whereas interchanging them gives the opposite effect.

In view of the fact that a size lens giving overall magnification magnifies in the horizontal meridian, it is, on purely geometrical grounds, surprising that it has little or no effect on one's orientation even in a " leaf room ", or on a tilting table, or other arrangements designed to discount the influence of experience and put stereopsis at a premium; in fact, overall size errors can be demonstrated only on arrangements designed to reveal image size disparities in different meridians separately.

The fact that an overall disparity has so little effect on one's orientation makes it less surprising that a vertical size difference has the same effect as a horizontal disparity but in the opposite direction. This, again, cannot be explained by theories based on simple geometrical projection.

Even more intriguing than the spatial distortions produced by these lenses are the sensations that they produce in normal subjects. A person walking about a grass lawn wearing a pair of meridional size lenses with their axes converging upwards or downwards will have the sensation that he is much smaller than usual and that he is wading through grass which offers no resistance to his passage. Alternatively, he may feel that he is far taller and yet that his feet scarcely reach the ground, according to which way the axes of the lenses converge. As their angular size is unchanged, daisies or flowers growing beside the lawn appear larger or smaller, according to whether they seem to be farther away or nearer. Grass with its abundance of detail is a particularly good testing ground, as the mind does not insist on its being flat as it does on the floor of a room being flat. That these sensations are pretty general is shown by the fact that at least half a dozen lay friends have independently described a pair of demonstration size lenses made up in a frame as " Alice Through the Looking Glass spectacles ".

Any optician can easily try these effects for himself with a trial frame and cylinders from his trial case.

The most interesting feature of these effects from the author's point of view is the time that they take to act. When setting a tilting table so as to appear level through oblique meridional size lenses, it is fully twenty seconds from the moment that he puts them on to the time that the table ceases to appear to move, and it is over a minute before he gets the maximum sensation on a grass lawn. A friend reports that one subject on whom he tried them got no effect for nearly ten minutes, but that she finally described her sensations as being as marked as anyone's.

In view of the fact that an overall size lens does cause discomfort, though it has little or no effect on one's spatial orientation, the writer prepared a stereo-card consisting of two circles approximately 30 and 31 mm. diameter, which gives a disparity of about 3 per cent. These are quite easily fused in an ordinary Holmes stereoscope, but looking at them for any length of time quickly produces a sense of marked discomfort. This figure was drawn at the necessary separation to reproduce the normal accommodation and convergence for 33 cm. when put in the stereoscope. With the larger circle to the left, all sense of discomfort was relieved by placing a pair of 15 $\triangle$ prisms in the lens cells of the instrument with their bases to the left. Putting them with their bases to the right greatly increased the sense of discomfort and even made fusion difficult. It will be noticed that the prisms allowed the eyes to turn in the direction in which the left eye could naturally get the larger image.

Most people who are interested in vision are familiar with the fact that flat prisms base-in will cause a flat surface to look convex, while prisms base-out make it look concave. This is generally attributed to the normal deviating power of the prism, but if the prisms are worked on a steep base curve the effect is greatly lessened, whereas if each eye is given a flat prism with a curved prism to neutralize its primary deviation this curving of flat surfaces is still seen. It is due to the fact that a flat prism possesses a small meridional magnifying power when looked through obliquely. It is possible to make a low power telescope out of two pairs of prisms arranged so that each pair magnifies cumulatively in its own meridian while the primary deviations and the chromatic dispersions cancel out, the two pairs of prisms being arranged with their base-apex lines at right angles to each other.

It seems clear that the curvature produced by prisms is due to an asymmetrical magnification effect and not to their interference with the subject's muscle balance.

CHAPTER V

THE EVIDENCE FROM ABNORMAL CONDITIONS

In addition to the experiments which we make in the laboratory there are those which nature makes for us which we can observe in the consulting room and clinic. Of these unfortunate people, those who suffer from chronic headaches seem to be the most instructive. Generally speaking, they fall into three classes, phoria cases, a few rare squint cases, and aniseikonia cases.

As we have already discussed the direct evidence that is offered by aniseikonia, all that we need to observe here is that as a cause of discomfort it is clinically indistinguishable from phorias, and that cases have been observed in which both defects could be demonstrated, and where the one which was responsible for the symptoms could be identified only by trial and error. In his limited experience of prescribing for aniseikonia, the author has known its correction give relief where the correction of an apparently significant phoria had failed, and he has also known the reverse occur, less often but only because the full correction of phorias should be tried before a size correction is ordered because it is a commoner source of trouble and the easier to provide a correction for.

We have already seen that it is difficult to define the position of rest of the eyes and this difficulty renders it equally difficult to put forward a rigid definition of a phoria. But the phoria situation is still further complicated by the fact that the visual axis of the eye appears not to be fixed relatively to the optical axis of the globe. Ames and Gliddon (4) have shown that if the eyes are presented with a pair of stereograms, such

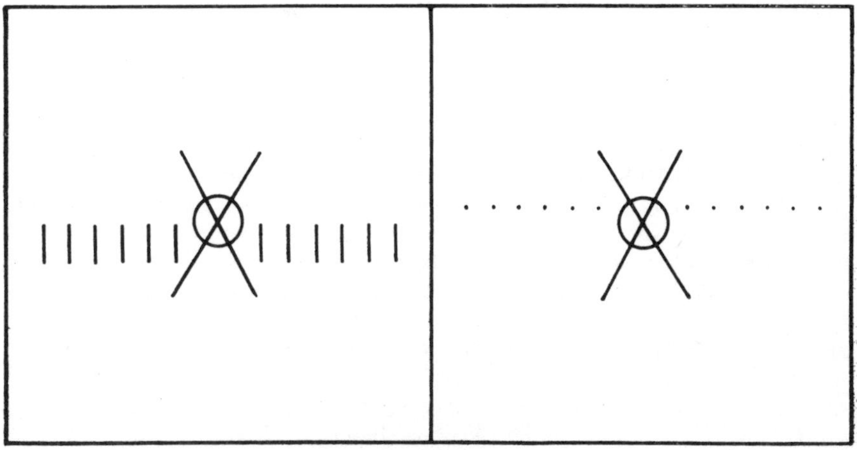

FIG. V 1.

as Fig. V, 1, where the central parts are fusible while the rest of the patterns are related but not identical, like a series of letters I on one side and their dots on the other, a displacement of the dots will be found in a large number of phoria cases, even though the central pattern was clearly fused. He also found that in two-thirds of the cases examined there was a close correlation between the prism required to place these dots in their correct position with respect to their I's and the phoria measured under conditions of dissociation. These cards also showed up vertical and cyclo phorias and some extreme cases of aniseikonia. It is of historical interest to notice that their discussion of the phenomena observed on these cards contains what appears to be the first germ of this important contribution to our knowledge of physiological optics.

The difficulty with this series of observations, as with most of those from the Dartmouth Eye Institute, and indeed almost all clinical establishments, is that the subjects were being investigated on account of symptoms which were believed to be due to their eyes and, as usual, a series of observations on subjects selected for the normality of their visual equipment is lacking.

They named this phenomena of the displacement of part of one uniocular image with respect to part of the other, while the parts common to both remained fused, " retinal slip ". The name " fixation disparity " has also been used in later papers. It is made use of empirically by quite a few opticians when they adjust a reading addition and even add prisms so as to equalise the lengths of the top and bottom arms of the E in the E x y z test. This should not be confused with Royce Warman's technique of using the top and bottom strokes of the z to balance the spherical elements of a correction (142a).

In studying the correlation between phoria measurements and retinal slip, Ames and Gliddon found that if the central locking target common to the two halves of the card were such as to show stereoscopic relief, the sense of depth appreciated by observers who showed no slip was greatly impaired if prisms were introduced to produce such a slip, while those who showed a slip in the first place found their appreciation of the depth in the central pattern improved when the slip was eliminated by prisms.

It seems clear that when slip is present the I's and their dots are falling on non-corresponding points, and that, consequently, the fusible patterns are also doing so and the subject is making use of his Panum's fusional areas in order to fuse the central pattern instead of bringing corresponding points to bear accurately. Ames and Gliddon, in their series of fifty-one cases, record five instances where patients who showed a near phoria of more than one metre angle but showed no retinal slip. In none of these cases did they find any reason to suppose that their phoria was the cause of their ocular discomfort.

The reduction in stereoscopic acuity which these workers have observed to accompany slip is particularly interesting as it seems to suggest that areas on opposite sides of the foveæ can, in some cases, act as corresponding points, while each fovea is brought into correspondence with a point still farther from the fovea. The resulting reduction of simultaneous acuity would, as Colenbrander (39) has shown, explain this loss in stereoscopic acuity and the correlation between poor stereo-acuity and large latent phorias manifested by the occlusion test which was noticed during the war (27) may also fit into this picture.

Another and perhaps more probable explanation of this reduction in stereoscopic acuity is that if eccentric points of Panum's areas are brought into correspondence the amount by which they overlap will be reduced and consequently the maximum disparity that may be fused without physiological diplopia occurring. This would have the effect of reducing the interval over which the mind performed its integration of disparities described in the next chapter.

The fact that it is possible to see points which do not lie on the same horopter in single simultaneous binocular vision is, of itself, a proof that non-corresponding retinal points can be fused under suitable circumstances, so the correlation between phoria measurements recorded by normal dissociation methods and the retinal slip cards in a variable prism stereoscope, and still more the cases where the correlation is not found, opens up a fascinating field for speculation and research.

Everyone who does any orthoptics has been surprised by cases who show large phorias which appear to cause them no distress. So far the writer knows of no measurement which distinguishes them from those who do suffer symptoms. The fact that Ames has found that in the few cases where he recorded a large phoria under dissociation, but none on the retinal slip method of measurement, the phoria did not appear to be the cause of the patient's symptoms, suggests that this may give us a means of telling whether a phoria is or is not to blame for a patient's symptoms without trying the effect of correcting it.

Such a test would have the further advantage that the ability to distinguish between a compensated and an uncompensated phoria would enormously simplify the recognition of an aniseikonia that required correction. Unfortunately, research into this is a clinical task and the experimenter is at the mercy of chance for the necessary subjects. A start has been made but progress is likely to be slow and it is unlikely that anything of value will have been achieved in time for inclusion in this essay.

Ames and Gliddon generally found that where there was a substantial difference between the dissociated phoria and the retinal slip reading, the latter was the smaller, but occasionally the reverse occurred. It may prove possible to correlate this with the results of the Marlow prolonged occlusion test.

Should it prove to be the case that a retinal slip measurement greater than the dissociation reading indicates that an occlusion test will reveal a phoria substantially greater than that which is immediately manifest, or if a zero slip reading indicates a fully compensated phoria, it would seem to suggest that ocular headaches are not always the result of sustaining a continuous innervation to the extraocular muscles, but of using a cortical mechanism designed for the evaluation of the significance of retinal disparities for the reconciliation of disparities which are not the result of the separation of the two eyes and therefore not significant to this evaluating mechanism, but which are due to imperfect convergence of the two eyes on the same point.

We saw in the last chapter that the eyes can fuse images which differ substantially in size, but that such fusion was accompanied by a sense of discomfort unless the mind was able to project them in a direction in which that size difference had some meaning for it. We now notice that when two unequal circles are being fused in a stereoscope the convergence cannot be equal to all points on their circumferences and that here too the mind must be using a cortical mechanism to supplement the extraocular muscles, as these can only produce one degree of convergence at a time. This supposition would explain why the symptoms of an uncompensated phoria and of aniseikonia are identical. That is what one would expect on this assumption, since both involve using this mechanism for a purpose for which it was not designed and in a manner which interferes with its performance of its correct function.

That a mechanism does exist which enables the brain to fuse disparate images is clearly demonstrated. That the use of this mechanism to fuse disparate images which are misleading can be the cause of discomfort seems to be proved both by clinical experience with aniseikonia patients and by some of the experiments in the last chapter. That it is the use of this mechanism to supplement convergence or divergence that gives rise to the symptoms of patients with uncompensated phorias is an unproved hypothesis. That this may be so, in a number of cases at least, seems to be likely when one considers the extreme similarity of the symptoms of uncompensated heterophoria and aniseikonia.

In the writer's experience, the patient who describes his spectacles as " drawing the eyes " or " making them feel that they are being dragged out ", is not a true phoria case, but has had his accommodation-convergence relationship upset by being given too strong a reading addition. Nevertheless, this patient has a phoria and is describing it in a manner which is typical of his class of case and not usual in aniseikonia cases. It may well be that his troubles are due to his frontal convergence reflex being suddenly called upon to do an amount of work to which it is not accustomed. It seems possible that such cases indicate that there are two radically distinct types of heterophoria differing in the manner in which they cause symptoms.

In considering symptoms from aniseikonia in support of this suggestion, it is important to remember that some degree of aniseikonia can be detected in the majority of people who are, none the less, free from all symptoms of binocular strain. Before accepting any explanation of the symptoms some of these patients suffer, it is necessary to explain why many people with the same defect do not have any symptoms at all. We may ignore small errors since, whatever the mechanism by which a defect causes distress, it is clear that a small enough defect will be tolerated, for no human being is absolutely symmetrical. Also the fact that a defect which is intolerable to one man is unnoticed by another is so well known as not to call for further comment. Clinically it is found that overall size errors cause least discomfort, while oblique meridional ones cause most, and horizontal meridional errors cause more distress than vertical ones, but less than oblique ones. This is the result that one would expect from the forms of spatial disorientation caused by an oblique error tilting the floor up or down, which seems more distressing than the lateral tilt produced by a horizontal discrepancy. A vertical discrepancy alone has no meaning for the mind, and when one is artificially produced the mind appears to apply the overall correction factor, and the disorientation produced is that associated with a horizontal size difference of the same sign in the other eye, though generally of somewhat less degree. We have seen that both horizontal and overall size differences have a meaning for the mind, even though it may have to reject that meaning; a vertical disparity has none, but it can be resolved into an overall component and a horizontal component. Ogle (109) has called this manifestation of a vertical error in one eye as a horizontal error in the other " the induced size effect ".

It is unusual for an aniseikonia patient to complain of spatial disorientation or to be conscious of it. It is often clearly demonstrable on the tilting table but the patient is usually as surprised by the demonstration as a normal individual is by the effect when imposed by size lenses. It appears that the mind applies a correction for the disorientation, the trouble manifests itself as headaches, or some other symptom. A curious fact that is sometimes noticed in patients who have reached middle age is that the mind appears to continue to apply this correction long after the need for it has been removed by optical means. The writer saw a patient recently who had worn size lenses for six months. On test she showed no signs of spatial disorientation and her headaches and other symptoms had completely gone, but she did still complain of some slight difficulty with space perception, though it was slowly passing off.

This should be compared with the complaints of disorientation which patients often make after a change in their spectacles. This also passes off, quickly in youth and less quickly in later life, so that in the fifties and sixties a change from toric to flat lenses and vice versa can cause considerable annoyance which may last a long time. These cases do not complain of headaches.

It seems that it is not the making of a mental allowance that causes headaches and eye strain, since these can be abolished by a correction long before the patient has grown sufficiently used to it to stop making an allowance which is no longer necessary, and it may be that this is one more instance where the misuse of Panum's areas may be the source of the discomfort. Their normal and proper use causes no distress and most people find that they can wear oblique size lenses indefinitely in comfort so long as they accept the resulting disorientation, but any effort to overcome it and to adapt themselves to their changed ocular conditions causes intense discomfort in a very short time. We see then that Panum's fusional areas may be employed to the full without discomfort and that a mental allowance for a non-existent disorientation can be made with no more discomfort than the resulting feeling of clumsiness, but that making an allowance in order to discount the evidence from retinal disparities can often cause discomfort.

The wearing of a size correction does not necessarily lead to any sense of disorientation even during the first few days. The writer recalls a patient who had never been able to read, sew, or watch a cinema in comfort, but who had no consciousness of spatial disorientation, yet a considerable oblique correction brought immediate relief of all her symptoms without causing even transitory secondary discomfort. This patient, a young married woman, was particularly interesting in that she was almost perfectly emmetropic. Her case history has been published by the writer (26).

As we noted above, it appears that the use of a considerable amount of retinal slip leads to a lowering of stereoscopic acuity. We also noted that there was some correlation between the results of a Marlow occlusion test and stereo-acuity (27), so it is interesting to recall the Navy found that it was uneconomical to attempt to train men with phorias of any size as stereoscopic range takers. The Air Force observations on the landing errors of pilots with phorias will be considered later.

We considered the oculo-motor reflexes in Chapter II and saw that their failure to become conditional in harmony with the refraction of the eye could lead to the development of strabismus. Chavasse considered all concomitant strabismus to be a perversion of the normal reflex development, arising from some circumstance causing clear vision to prove a greater reward than single binocular vision, as may be expected in cases with unusually large hypermetropic errors.

In a child with 6 dioptres of hypermetropia who wishes to see clearly at 25 centimetres, 10 dioptres of accommodation are needed while the convergence normally associated with 4 dioptres only is called for. It is not surprising that such cases often break down into a squint. That this is, in many cases, the mechanism of the breakdown is proved by the fact that correcting the hypermetropia alone will often cure the squint, provided that no time is lost, but that it is not the whole story is obvious from the facts that almost all children are born hypermetropic, that most of those who continue hypermetropic into adult life have no squint and that many which do break down have no more than the normal hypermetropia for their age.

Very many of these cases break down during the course of some childish ailment, whooping-cough being the most notable offender. Chavasse (36) suggested that the probable mechanism was some passing toxic paresis of one or more extraocular muscles, but it seems just as likely that it may be the result of an abnormal stimulation of the tone of their antagonists. That such a stimulation to convergence is possible is shown by the sudden transitory squint seen in an infant afflicted with wind.

An increase of tone of the two medial recti during an illness could be the result of some direct stimulation, or of the release of some lower centre from cortical inhibition (2). It seems likely, from the experiments of Powell (112) and Colson (40) that the latter is the explanation in the case of the increase in esophoria and occasional esotropia that results from the excessive use of alcohol, particularly in view of the observation that alcohol may have some therapeutic use in the treatment of amblyopia (12). The fact that the eyes normally diverge before a full surgical anæsthesia is reached suggests that the temporary selective weakening of one set of muscles compared to another from toxic causes is quite possible.

Yet many hypermetropic children have whooping cough, measles, and the whole gamut of children's ailments without developing a squint. This, among other considerations, led Worth (154) to postulate a defect of the fusion faculty as a necessary condition for the development of a squint in addition to an abnormal convergence of the visual axes. Chavasse

(36) did not agree with this view, but held that all squints should be regarded as perversion of the normal binocular reflexes resulting from obstacles operating during the development of the reflexes.

The writer (34) has found that alcohol causes a marked reduction of fusional reserves, so it seems at least possible that the reason that so many children start a squint during an attack of whooping cough or measles is that the infections cause a specific intoxication which produces the same effect. Where the phorias were small and the powers of fusion adequate, no harm would be done, but where there was an excessive amount of hypermetropia associated with poor fusional reserves a squint might well result.

There are many possible obstacles to the normal development of fusion which Chavasse classifies under the headings: sensory, motor, and central. Motor obstacles are of no interest for the present discussion. It is obvious that if the two eyes form images which differ greatly in clarity, size, or shape, the brain will have greater difficulty in fusing them than if they were well matched. That children with markedly different refraction in the two eyes are more prone to squints than those with equal refraction is too well known to need further comment. Though no observations on the point have been made in this country, there is a certain amount of evidence from America that a proportion of squinters show marked degrees of aniseikonia, so that it too must be considered among the possible obstacles to fusion. It is possible that it is the explanation of the horror fusionis observed in certain cases which we will be considering shortly.

Lyle (97) lists as central causes hystero-malingering, physical or mental trauma, hyper- or hypo-excitability of the central nervous system and, as a possibility, central monocular inhibition. It will be noticed that in this list he does not include any congenital lack or weakness of the fusion faculty, although he does, at a later stage, mention that there are certain cases where the ability to fuse seems wholly wanting.

The markedly hereditary character of squint seems to lend support to the idea that in some families the fusion reflex is slow to develop, if not actually defective, but against this must be set the fact that in none of the cases that the writer has seen where fusion appeared to be impossible was there any family history of strabismus.

He has now seen three cases of manifest strabismus where he was quite unable to demonstrate any reason for the patient's failure to fuse; all three were alternators with full normal visual acuity in each eye and each, with the necessary refractive correction, had a muscle balance well within normal limits after a short period of monocular occlusion. One case which was investigated in great detail will be described as representative of the three. She is a married woman, aged 25, with about 5·0 D of hypermetropia in each eye. She sought advice for the relief of daily, crippling headaches. When first seen she had a manifest convergent alternating squint of approximately five degrees. As her spectacles corrected her small amount of astigmatism accurately, that was ruled out as a possible cause of her headaches. On attempting to measure the angle of the deviation more accurately with prisms and a torch, the angle increased steadily as prisms were added, until suddenly the eye swung outwards and remained relatively deviating until the prism power had been reduced to one or two prism dioptres. Subsequently, on a synoptophore she went from about twenty degrees convergent to about five to ten divergent in order to evade fusion. No signs of abnormal retinal correspondence could be demonstrated either with the synoptophore, or with the after-image test. In order to see whether her headaches were due to her eyes she was advised to do a week's monocular occlusion. Her headaches stopped completely and immediately on removing the occluder her eyes were seen to be straight, but almost immediately one eye turned inwards to the original angle. After a further week's occlusion she was found to be orthophoric both horizontally and vertically at six metres, and a very unsteady reading of about 2△ of esotropia at 33 cm. was obtained with the Maddox wing. No cyclophoria could be found and with the Lancaster red-green lanterns and diplopia goggles she showed perfect orthophoria at one metre in all directions of gaze.

The age of onset of the squint was given as less than two years and she had an idea that it may have been much earlier. The headaches started before she was eleven and had got progressively worse. As there was no fusion, it was impossible to make any measurements for aniseikonia and orthoptics were impossible; so as there was no muscular defect that could be operated on she was advised to continue occlusion as a therapeutic measure in the hope that later it might prove possible to train her to fuse.

The interest in this and other similar cases lies in the fact that she has preserved almost perfect orthophoria and a normal convergence-accommodation relationship in the absence of fusion. There is no evidence that she has ever suffered any form of oculo-motor paresis, and yet there is an active avoidance of fusion.

Before considering the possible implications of this case, one very similar should be mentioned. Here also the patient was a woman, aged 29, who was troubled by daily headaches. Her refraction was also about + 5·0 D, and when seen she had a manifest alternating divergent squint of 15°. As a child she had had a convergent squint and could still be made into a convergent squinter by reducing her plus correction. Her muscle balance and accommodation-convergence relationship were, again, well within normal limits, the essential difference between her and the others was that I was able to locate the obstacle to fusion, namely, a cyclotropia of 15°. Despite the fact that she appeared to be perfectly concomitant now, it is possible that this was paretic in origin, though the fact that her eyes remained straight under indefinite occlusion makes me think it improbable. Even when the cyclotropia was allowed for on a synoptophore she had no fusion.

This case was described fully in a paper that the author read at the London Refraction Hospital Silver Jubilee Convention (30), together with two somewhat similar cases. The previous case is reported here for the first time. At the time the author suggested the name " purposive strabismus " for them, having overlooked the fact that Chavasse had already used the term to describe squints of similar ætiology, but which had become incorporated into the normal reflex tonus of the muscles and so do not vanish under occlusion. He now prefers to call them " evasion squints " from their similarity to the vertical evasion sometimes seen when squinters with fusion difficulties are approaching parallelism under orthoptic training that Mein has described (102).

Lyle (97) has pointed out that imitative squints and the squints produced by children from curiosity never become permanent in the absence of a latent deviation. It appears that these evasion squints are similar in that they have never become permanent for lack of the necessary latent deviation. The obstacle to fusion compels the patient to maintain the deviation constantly in order to separate the two images, but this innervation has not become conditional and part of the reflex tonus of the muscles, so the deviation is maintained in just the same way as a phoria patient overcomes his latent deviation in the interests of fusion. Here again we have a squint due to a perversion of a normal reflex, but it is the fusion reflex and not a convergence reflex which has become perverted. Their headaches are, presumably, due to the sustained abnormal innervation.

This second case also raises the question of whether there is, or is not, a divergence centre in the brain, or whether need to evade fusion can cause an innervation from occipital sources, just as the need for fusion seems to do, though it must be admitted that fifteen degrees of divergence seems surprisingly large, especially when we remember that a very similar case only used five degrees of convergence. However, this may well be connected with the fact that the patient who diverged had never completely lost diplopia.

Another similar case where the deviation started with measles at the age of six months so that the patient could never have developed any binocular vision worthy of the name retained an almost normal accommodation-convergence relationship and orthophoria with her refraction corrected and one eye occluded. She had some five degrees of cyclophoria and maintained a five degree convergent squint, but luckily did not suffer much discomfort.

Since this chapter was written, the author has had the good fortune of seeing one of these evasion squints in such an early stage of development that it has proved possible to reverse the process of development. The patient was a girl of eighteen who had lived in the Highlands until a few months before, when she had come to London in order to enter domestic service. Up till then she had believed that her eyesight was perfect and she had certainly been quite free of symptoms.

Soon after coming to London she began to suffer from slight headaches. As a consequence she was refracted and prescribed R.E. + 0·50 cyl. axis 35°; L.E. − 7·00 sph. − 2·75° cyl. axis 25°. At this stage she was orthophoric at distance and showed a small exophoria at near. As the left eye was somewhat amblyopic she was advised to cover the right eye and use the left when reading. She quickly achieved rather better than 6/9 corrected acuity in this eye and, equally soon, she began to suffer from crippling headaches.

She was referred to the author who found a 5° divergent strabismus. He accordingly prescribed a frosted lens for the left eye and awaited results. After six weeks she reported that all her symptoms had subsided and her muscle balance was again normal; she was then given a plano lens for her left eye.

It seems clear that the original headaches, concerning which she sought advice, were due solely to the small degree of hyperopic astigmatism in her right eye. She still cannot dispense comfortably with its correction. The manifest squint that she had when the writer first saw her must have been due to the size difference between two clear images making them unfusible. The author hopes, later, to be able to give her at least a partial correction for her refractive error and image size difference.

These cases are strong evidence for the correctness of Chavasse's contention that the basic occipital accommodation-convergence reflex is unconditional and innate. On the question of the possibility of a congenital defect of the fusion faculty they are less helpful. In one, the presence of an adequate obstacle to fusion was demonstrated, namely her cyclotropia. However, in view of the results of the author's experiments on occlusion, reported in Chapter II, this may have been the result of the dissociation of her two eyes and not the cause of it. In the third case, the history suggests that though no adequate obstacle could be proved to be still operating, binocular vision may well have been interrupted by some transitory paresis at so early an age that a normal fusion reflex may have been perverted into horror fusionis. The first case described seems, on the face of it, the best evidence for an innate defect of the fusion faculty since no obstacle to binocular vision can be demonstrated and, as we shall see later, there are reasonable grounds for thinking that she has never suffered from any form of oculo-motor paresis. Her hypermetropia is very considerable and such as might readily lead to a typical Donders' squint, but in the absence of some defect of the power of fusion it is difficult to see why she did not regain binocular vision on having spectacles prescribed in early childhood. Unfortunately, it proved impossible to get accurate dates for the onset of the squint, or the date at which spectacles were first prescribed.

Giles (64) quotes a case of Hawkes' of a squinter with a comparatively trifling amount of hypermetropia in each eye who had responded well to orthoptic treatment at first but could achieve fusion only when the acuity of one eye was reduced to 6/12 by over-correction. Peripheral fusion appeared easy to obtain, but the macular fusion of two clear images was impossible.

Bannon (10) holds the view that some weakness of the fusion faculty is a necessary condition for the occurrence of a concomitant squint, but that it is not sufficient to cause one by itself. That the fusion faculty is a separate entity quite distinct from bi-fixation and is cortical is proved both by Winkelmann's flicker experiments described in Chapter II, and by Ames' retinal slip experiments described in this chapter. Fusion is clearly reflex and therefore, unless unconditional, it requires reinforcing by some reward. If, as seems to the writer likely, this reflex is nearing becoming unconditional, its strength and the reinforcement needed to consolidate it might easily vary from family to family, and individual to individual. If so, some obstacle to fusion which would be trivial to one subject might be sufficient to disrupt binocular vision permanently in another.

It seems reasonable to believe that a congenital weakness of the fusion faculty is possible, but unnecessary to believe in the possibility of its absence, or in congenital horror fusionis. The first of these three cases that I have described is the most perfect one that the writer knows of to support the congenital horror fusionis theory, but he is still hoping that it may prove possible to measure some aniseikonia in her at some later date, and that it may finally prove possible to teach her to fuse.

The diagnostic feature which is pathognomonic of these evasion squints is that the headaches and asthenopic symptoms of which they complain are immediately relieved by monocular occlusion, and that this relief is accompanied by a reduction in the angle of deviation. As we noticed in Chapter II, Marlow introduced the use of monocular occlusion as a diagnostic measure in grief cases where he suspected that the cause might be a phoria which was not immediately manifest. The Dartmouth Eye Institute extended its range and used it as a test of whether a patient's symptoms were, or were not, due to some binocular anomaly. Both they and the present writer have found it a most valuable guide to the likelihood of relieving a patient's symptoms by an aniseikonic prescription. In addition, both they and some clinics at the London Refraction Hospital have found it a most valuable aid in the prescription of prisms and the treatment of phorias.

In the course of some experiments done on volunteers from the recent full-time second year course at the Northampton Polytechnic and a few others, where phorias were recorded at regular intervals, one or two abnormal cases were found. One student went from 2 △ eso to 12 △ eso in twenty-four hours, so he was told to stop the test; another, after five days of right occlusion, during which he had drifted from 1 △ eso to 2 △ eso and 2 △ right hyperphoria, suddenly swung to 11 △ eso, 6 △ right hyperphoria, 14 △ of excyclophoria.

It is interesting to compare these results with those of the prism-provoked diplopia test described by Sédan and Sédan-Bauby (123), where they show that on forcing diplopia by means of a prism for a considerable period, on removing the prism the subject takes far longer to recover binocular vision than normally if the prism had made an extra call on a muscle that had once suffered a paresis. The fact that both these students experienced diplopia for some hours—the second for nearly twelve hours—suggests an affinity between the tests. It is difficult to suggest any other explanation for this sudden change in the muscle balance of a subject selected for the apparent normality of his binocular vision and for his return to his normal muscle balance inside twenty-four hours, when no sign of phoria or paresis would be found with Lancaster's red and green lanterns.

These sudden changes in the direction of esophoria in selected normal young adults are extremely difficult to explain except on the basis of the dying away of tonus which has become almost incorporated in the normal ocular reflexes through the long sustained innervation necessary to compensate for some old paresis. It is easy but important to differentiate between these instances and those met with normally in clinical practice. These were chosen as symptom free and returned to being symptom free inside twenty-four hours. Clinical cases are selected because they have symptoms which may be due to some binocular cause, but which may not. If the cause is some binocular anomaly, it is uncompensated. For this reason, it is essential when experimenting on young and apparently normal subjects to take daily readings of their muscle balances, as any anomaly that they may show is fully compensated. Twenty-four hours of the changed condition is not likely to upset their compensation, but ten days might do so.

Considerable swings in the direction of increased exophoria are, as we have seen, quite common in normal subjects, and Marlow's (98) explanation that they are due to a reversion to an earlier evolutionary state is quite possible. However, it seems more likely to the writer that they show that the tonus to maintain parallelism is not as yet fully conditioned. In the cases who exhibit symptoms which are relieved by occlusion, it is likely that a considerable part at least of the change is due to a relaxing of an innervation which should more properly be called a state of spasm than of tonus, in view of the number of people whose muscle balance shows little change, even after three weeks of complete dissociation.

Extending the observations of Powell and of Colson recorded above, while he has confirmed that alcohol tends to reduce exophoria and increase esophoria, the writer cannot find that it has any effect on hyperphoria and little, if any, on the accommodation-convergence relationship. He does find that it leads to a marked decrease in the amount of vertical prism that can be overcome without diplopia being observed. It therefore seems probable that the diplopia sometimes experienced by subjects under the influence of alcohol is due, not so much to the esophoria induced but by the reduced power of the fusion reflex to overcome it. The reason for this is not immediately obvious since alcohol appears to act chiefly by the reduction of central inhibitions, but in view of similarity between some of the symptoms of alcoholic intoxication and fever, it seems at least possible that this is the method by which such illnesses as whooping cough and measles precipitate a squint in childhood. It is also possible that alcohol produces diplopia by a process of releasing an inhibition of the first cells in the cortex which the visual impulses reach.

Two years ago the writer saw a case with Mr. D. W. A. Mitchell at the London Refraction Hospital. She was a woman of about thirty; one eye was emmetropic but the other was myopic by more than 20 D and, though it appeared perfectly healthy, could not be corrected to better than about 4/60; its fixation was so poor that it was impossible to get any muscle balance, but the eyes appeared to be perfectly straight. She reported that until about three years previously she had believed the eye to be blind. About that time she began to be conscious that the eye had some measure of sight and began to experiment with it for herself. She achieved a certain amount of deneutralization and from that time on suffered from almost continuous headaches and pain round that eye; until then she had been perfectly comfortable.

This was during the period that the author was introducing the occlusion test at the Refraction Hospital, but he did not consider that the eye had sufficient vision to cause any trouble and was of the opinion that either her headaches were not of ocular origin, or that there was some pathological condition that he had failed to detect. Mr. Mitchell also could detect no signs of any pathological condition, and pointed out that if there was one it had remained stationary for nearly three years, so that there could scarcely be any hurry over referring her for further investigation, so he decided to try the effect of a fortnight's occlusion. For reasons of hospital convenience she then passed under his care. When she next reported all her original symptoms had disappeared. It is perhaps worth recording, as a warning to those who contemplate using the occlusion test, that she complained of a new set of pains over the other eye which proved to be due to an unduly tight elastic on the eye shade that she was wearing. As the eye was functionally useless, at least so long as she retained the sight of the other, we prescribed an opaque contact lens for which she has an excellent tolerance.

A year later she was still comfortable and reported that so long as she kept that eye occluded she had no headaches, but that ten minutes' exposure sufficed to start one which might take as much as two days to disappear completely. That this was a binocular effect is shown by the fact that half an hour's exposure of her bad eye with the good eye occluded causes no discomfort.

It is difficult to explain why so poor a percept as her cortex receives from that eye can cause so much trouble. One can only suppose that she must have a very excellent cortical binocular mechanism, and that having in the past broken down her suppression, her brain tries to make use of unusable signals. Very similar effects are sometimes seen when partial occlusion is attempted. As a concession to a patient's vanity, the author has, in the past, occasionally used a frosted lens as an occluder for diagnostic purposes. On several occasions the patient has returned saying that the headaches had been much worse, and that the experiment had proved unbearable, yet when the patient was persuaded to try again but with total occlusion, the result was complete comfort.

Roper and Bannon (118) reported a case of Dr. W. B. Lancaster's where he prescribed an opaque contact lens for a young woman who suffered continuous headaches after a burn in the neighbourhood of the macula from seeing the sun reflected in a concave mirror that she was polishing. After some months of comfort her headaches suddenly returned. The explanation proved to be that a small portion of the enamel used to render the lens opaque had chipped off and that a small amount of peripheral light was entering her eye, though not enough for her to appreciate that it was seeing anything. Her symptoms disappeared again immediately the fault was rectified.

Somewhere between these cases and the evasion squints lie those unfortunate strabismus cases, generally young adults, who were perfectly comfortable until some practitioner broke down their suppression before discovering that he could not give them fusion. Mercifully, they are fairly uncommon though not nearly so rare as they should be. The diplopia in these cases is usually the chief complaint and it is an unfortunate fact that once suppression has been overcome patients generally recover it only with great difficulty.

We noticed when discussing retinal slip that retinal correspondence is by no means rigid, as indeed is obvious from the fact that, within limits, single binocular vision of points of different parallax is possible. Certain squint patients show a condition which seems to be an extension of this effect known as abnormal retinal correspondence. In his condition some degree of fusion is possible at an angle other than the angle of deviation. The difference between the angle at which fusion can be elicited in a haploscope and the angle of deviation is known as the angle of anomaly, if the angle of anomaly is equal to the angle of deviation the abnormal correspondence is said to be harmonious, and the patient will be found to have some degree of binocular vision while squinting; for instance, he will probably see the two coloured cards in a Remy separator simultaneously and side by side. If the two angles are not equal the correspondence is said to be inharmonious, and no sort of binocular vision is possible without instrumental aid.

Where a harmonious abnormal retinal correspondence exists the binocular vision must necessarily be low grade, since the macula of one eye is being brought into correspondence with a point some ten degrees or more from the macula of the other eye, and the visual acuity of that point will be low. Abnormal retinal correspondence, when well established, can be a most formidable obstacle to the cure of strabismus, and cases have been recorded where it has caused a reversion to the original deviation after an apparently successful operation. Chavasse (36) has described cases where monocular diplopia and binocular quadriplopia have occurred during the cure of abnormal correspondence.

Before considering the probable mechanism of this phenomenon, it is essential to stress the difference between it and false projection. The latter is a monocular effect, normally associated with deep amblyopia of the fixing eye, often with false fixation, where long misuse has caused a change of local sign to occur. Abnormal retinal correspondence is a binocular effect and, in the writer's experience, though opinion is not unanimous on this point, most often found in alternators; it is certainly seen in its most highly developed form only in them. Here each eye retains perfect fixation with full visual acuity and, by itself, normal projection; the anomaly can be demonstrated only when the two eyes are associated. The most convincing demonstration is Bielchowsky's after-image test. The subject, with one eye covered, fixates a black spot in the middle of the glowing filament of a strip light held vertically for about ten seconds. The lamp is extinguished and the procedure is repeated on the other eye, with the light held horizontally for a similar period. The subject is then told to close his eyes and inspect the after-images that he sees. As soon as he is clear as to the figure formed by the two after-images, he is given paper and pencil and told to draw them. A normal subject will draw a perfectly symmetrical cross, but a subject with well developed abnormal correspondence will draw a figure like the letter T lying on its side with, perhaps, some overlap of the horizontal stroke, or a gap between it and the upright, depending on the angle of anomaly and the geometry of the test.

Since there is no false projection, it is clear that the two maculæ, when used together, have ceased to be corresponding points and that some new system of binocular retinal correspondence has been built up. This is confirmed by the fact that fusion can be demonstrated in a haploscope at the anomalous angle. Many workers have claimed to have found stereopsis of sorts in these cases when fusing at the angle of anomaly; others have denied it. Duke-Elder (50 *a*) sums up against it. The writer is disposed to the view that " it all depends on what you mean by stereopsis "; if there is any form of bifixation with convergence one would expect to find such a degree of stereopsis as a hand three needle test can show, and on his view of the mechanism of the anomaly, some degree of disparity stereopsis could be possible, but the low acuity of the anomalously corresponding area must, of necessity, cause either form of stereopsis, particularly disparity stereopsis, to be very poor. However, most of the experienced orthoptists that the author has asked are quite convinced that it is sometimes present.

We noticed in the first chapter that interconnections within the occipital cortex are effected by relays of short neurons, and we saw from our retinal slip experiments in the last chapter that correspondence is flexible, even in normal subjects. It is possible with a variable prism stereoscope to show that points as much as 15′ on either side of normal may be brought into correspondence, but there is no sense of the fused target having moved; it is only the points seen monocularly which are therefore being projected normally which seem to move. We have, then, the situation that part of each retina is projecting normally, and the part which is serving binocular vision is projecting abnormally in the interests of fusion.

Remembering that cells stimulated by corresponding points in each eye are closely intermingled in the cortex, it seems necessary to suppose that projection is not always as from the cells immediately stimulated from the lateral geniculates, but from cells which receive their impulses from those first cells, but after one or more relays. Fusion must be a process of finding a cell accessible to the two cells first stimulated, such that it can respond to both of them simultaneously.

We shall develop some of the possibilities of that idea further in the next chapter. It is introduced here as it seems to the writer that abnormal retinal correspondence is an extension of that flexibility of fusion which is normally confined to Panum's areas. It must be that long association of areas which do not normally correspond has by repeated stimulation opened up an association pathway, through a long chain of synapses, which has led to the inhibition of the normal correspondence. That there must be an active inhibitory mechanism is obvious, as without it the rotation of the eyes, as produced in the retinal slip experiments, would lead to immediate diplopia instead of continued fusion and single vision of objects whose images fell on non-corresponding points would be impossible. Physiological diplopia would be the normal state and not a trick that one learns.

It might be thought at first sight that if this were so, a squinter with equal acuity in each eye would project from the binoculus and split the angle of deviation between his eyes. However, the loss of acuity resulting renders this an unstable state, and the lower acuity of the abnormally corresponding area produces the effect demonstrated with plus lenses and neutral filters of transferring the centre of projection from one eye to the other (28). If this is accepted, alternators with abnormal retinal correspondence do not differ from those without for the purposes of our next question.

This next problem is: How do alternators maintain two accurate systems of projection and sensory correspondence? The author regards this as further evidence that the extraocular muscles have no important proprioception. Innervations for voluntary eye movements, eye movements which are originated by a stimulus at a conscious level, are reported to appropriate centres of the brain in order to stabilise the visual field. Movements originated at lower levels, such as convergence, are not. One can initiate convergence voluntarily, but only by the exercise of one's imagination. The imagining of a nearby point of attention is voluntary, but the resulting convergence is reflex. If one adducts one eye, with the other eye occluded by a lateral version, the surrounding scene does not seem to move; if one makes the same movement of the eye by converging on an imaginary object, the surroundings do move. The movements that an alternator makes when changing eyes are involuntary, and as such would produce a sense of movement in his surroundings, were it not that as he changes eyes he also changes his point of projection and reverses his central inhibitions, so that the same projection cells postulated above are being stimulated as before.

This is not always true of paretic alternators; the writer saw one recently whose chief complaint was that she was continually losing her place when reading. Watching her it became clear that this occurred regularly when she alternated. She was not aware that she had a squint as it was cosmetically insignificant.

It seems reasonable to suppose that inharmonious abnormal retinal correspondence was originally harmonious, but that the angle of deviation has changed either too quickly for the correspondence to keep pace, or too late for a fresh one to be built up.

CHAPTER VI

BINOCULAR SPACE PERCEPTION

Woodworth (151) describes the school of Gestalt psychology as holding that the individual's process of learning, perceiving, and thinking is always a process of working from the whole to the part, and not a process of summing parts to make a whole. I have to confess that my own sympathies lie more with the Behaviourist school, in that I am loath to attach any great weight to evidence gleaned from introspection. In considering visual space, one is forced to admit that preconceptions of the Gestalt can exercise a determining influence on what we see. In the previous chapters we have noticed several instances of this, the mind's refusal to accept a landscape which is being moved to and fro by optical means and its insistence that it is the stationary reference mark which moves. The difficulty of appreciating artificial pseudoscopy of familiar objects and, perhaps most significant, the congruent rooms constructed by Ames.

The great interest and importance of these congruent rooms lies in the fact that they demonstrate the great difference that is possible between the physical stimulus and what two eyes see; a room without a straight line or flat surface in it may be seen as a normal rectangular room, larger or smaller than the physical reality according to whether the sides of this are concave or convex.

It is clear that some preconception of the pattern of the whole is needed to enable the mind to erect a percept which differs fundamentally from the physical object which provided the stimulus, but this perception cannot result solely from a process of working from the whole to the part. In order that it shall be possible to perceive these different rooms as congruent, it is necessary that they shall bear a certain mathematical relationship to each other. A line element dx_1, dy_1, dz_1, of one and the corresponding line element dx_2, dy_2, dz_2 of the other must be such that $d\gamma_1 = d\gamma_2$, $d\phi_1 = d\phi_2$ and $d\theta_1 = d\theta_2$ where γ is the binocular parallax, ϕ binocular latitude and θ the angle of elevation. It can only be by working from the part to the whole in a situation where the data can bear more than one interpretation that the mind can have the freedom to select the solution that fits best into a preconceived pattern.

With this introduction the writer proposes to attempt a description of Luneburg's mathematical analysis of binocular vision (96) so far as possible, in non-mathematical language. The first point to insist on is that this analysis is a mathematical description of subjective space as experiment shows it to be; it does not attempt to explain why it is so. The next few pages are an attempt to show in outline what Luneburg did and his justification for doing it. So far as possible, points will be dealt with in the order in which he took them; for a fuller treatment the reader is referred to the original monograph.

The first necessity is to justify the idea of applying mathematical treatment to subjective sensations. To do this it is necessary to be able to co-ordinate sensations by numbers. It may be that some psychological manifolds are not capable of numerical treatment; Luneberg shows, however, that visual space is. Considering first the one-dimensional manifold of height, Luneburg shows that if it is possible to say of three height sensations, S_1, S_2, S_3, that, if S_3 is greater than S_2, which in turn is greater than S_1, and further that, if the contrast ($S_2\, S_3$) is greater than the contrast ($S_1\, S_2$) then the psychometric co-ordination of numbers to sensations within the manifold is uniquely determined with the sole reservation that there remains an arbitrary scale factor, which means that only relative size, not absolute size, is determined, and that the origin of the scale is also undetermined. He then proceeds to show that if this is true of a one-dimensional manifold it is also true of a three-dimensional one.

The metric for a manifold of points is defined as the rule for measuring objects in that manifold, and it is sufficient to formulate that rule for " infinitesimally " small objects in order to define the manifold. Considering two points on a piece of graph paper whose Cartesian co-ordinates differ by dx and dy, we know from Pythagoras that their separation $ds = \sqrt{dx^2 + dy^2}$ or $ds^2 = dx^2 + dy^2$, the metric of the Euclidean plane from which the whole of Euclidean geometry may be developed by analytical methods.

The problem of proceeding from the infinitesimally small to the finite is the problem of choosing the shortest of all the possible curves joining two points of the manifold. Its length is obtained by summing its elements and it is uniquely determined by the condition that this integral shall be a minimum. Such a unique curve in any manifold is called a geodesic. The geodesic in the Euclidean plane is the straight line and, in the case of two points S apart, it is defined by $S = \int\sqrt{dx^2 + dy^2} =$ minimum or in Euclidean space $S = \int\sqrt{dx^2 + dy^2 + dz^2} =$ minimum.

Its simplicity and long familiarity have led most of us to think of Euclidean space as the only possible space, and even of the Euclidean plane as the typical surface; yet the surface of the globe is not a Euclidean plane and cannot even be mapped on one without distortion. To project the surface of a sphere onto a sheet of paper wrapped round it in a cylinder whose axis coincides with the reference axis of the sphere, we need a piece of paper whose width is equal to the circumference of the sphere, but the two lines of that same length which represent the two poles would fall off the paper however long it was. This form of projection, Mercator's, is used for many charts and in the neighbourhood of the equator is most satisfactory. As you near the poles distances get exaggerated and shapes distorted; its convenience lies in the fact that directions remain unchanged. If you draw a straight line joining two points on a Mercator's chart, measure the angle that it makes with the meridian and use that bearing as your course in sailing from point to the other, you will reach your destination. But unless one point lies due north of the other, or both are on the equator, you will not have gone the shortest way. The metric of the chart is not the metric of the globe, and so the geodesic of the one is not the geodesic of the other. The geodesics of a sphere are " great circles ", circles which pass through opposite ends of a diameter. In Mercator's projection the only great circles which are represented by straight lines are the equator and the circles of longitude, which pass through the two poles. The metric of a unit sphere is $ds^2 = dx^2 + \sin^2 x \, . \, dy^2$.

This instance of a two-dimensional non-Euclidean geometry has been dealt with at some length because it is easy to follow, and once the existence of non-Euclidean geometries of two dimensions have been grasped it is easier to accept the extension of the idea to three or more dimensions, even though the great majority of people find it impossible to visualise such a space. This is not surprising in view of the fact that the geodesic of visual space must be presented to consciousness as a straight line.

We know that we can accept physical space as Euclidean to a sufficiently close approximation for all our purposes in such limited regions as concern binocular vision. If then we compare the geodesics of our visual space, its apparent straight lines, with those of Euclidean space, we shall at least get a clue to its metric.

Enough has probably been said to make it clear that there are an infinite number of possible non-Euclidean geometries, and it is necessary to ask whether they are all possible for our visual space. Luckily they are not. We know that we regard the form and the position of objects as independent. It is a psychological conviction to each one of us that a rigid body will retain its size and shape when moved from one portion of space to another. The movability of rigid objects is, then, one of the conditions which the psychometric of visual space must fulfil. It is true that a change of spectacles often produces temporary distortions of objects as they move, and that such distortions are easily produced with size lenses, but it is a psychological necessity to neutralize these distortions even at the cost of crippling headaches or the total suppression of binocular vision, so it is right to accept movability as a condition for visual space and this condition is fulfilled only by a very limited class of geometries, the geometries of constant curvature. Euclidean geometry is the special case of zero curvature while the surface of a sphere has a two-dimensional geometry of constant positive curvature.

In a previous chapter we noticed that when a subject was asked to arrange upright rods, or other suitable targets, so that they should lie in a frontal plane, if all clues other than those from binocular vision were excluded, there was only one distance at which he placed them in a Euclidean straight line, and then only in the central region. Within that distance he would place them in a curve concave towards him; beyond it the curve would have its convex side towards him. To the subject these curves appear to be straight horizontal lines at right angles to his median plane. To the outside observer with instrumental facilities at his disposal they are not straight. They are not geodesics in Euclidean space, but since he sees them as straight they are geodesics in the visual space of the subject.

When Blumenfeld (19) repeated Hillebrand's alley experiments he found that to tell the subject to arrange successive pairs of targets so as to be equidistant on either side of the median plane, is not the same to the subject as telling him to arrange them in two straight lines parallel to it.

We may, for brevity, call one arrangement the equidistant alley and the other the parallel alley.

In Euclidean geometry parallel lines remain equidistant from each other. This is not so in other geometrics, it is, in fact, the distinguishing feature of Euclidean geometry. It is possible to reconstruct the whole of it from this condition by geometrical means, just as it is possible to do so from its metric, $ds^2 = dx^2 + dy^2$, by analytical methods. In Euclidean geometry the two instructions to the subject, to form an equidistant alley or to form a parallel alley, are identical and if the subject's visual space were Euclidean he would not distinguish between them. But he does make such a distinction and is consistent about it. Both alleys have curved sides in Euclidean space, and if the farthest pair of points is common to both, the rest of the parallel alley lies consistently within the equidistant alley. Since the subject has made the sides of the parallel alley straight lines, they are, like the horopters, geodesics of his visual space.

We have seen that visual space must be a space of constant curvature, since size and location are independent. It is not Euclid's space of zero curvature since its geodesics are not in general, straight lines in Euclidean space. This last observation that the parallel alley lies within the equidistant alley shows that it is a space of constant negative curvature, Lobachevski's hyperbolic geometry.

Two straight trumpets with widely flared mouths joined together would form a close approximation to a surface of constant negative curvature. As it has much in common with the surface of a sphere, such a surface has been called a pseudosphere. Since it is less familiar than a sphere and more difficult to visualise, it is even less help than the sphere in any attempt that one may make to visualise a curved space. Such attempts are, luckily, useless since the important thing about one's subjective space is that its geodesics are, to oneself, straight lines. The " model " that one constructs for one's self of one's own subjective space is Euclidean space. Poincaré, the great French mathematician (not to be confused with the politician) devised a " model " of such a space which is helpful to us, namely an optical medium of refractive index $n = \frac{1}{1 - \rho^2}$, where ρ is a function of the distance from the origin. It can be pictured as a series of concentric spherical layers round the origin, each of greater refractive index than the one inside it. Light rays in such a medium would follow paths like the geodesics of visual space.

Surveying instruments in such a space would survey a space of constant negative curvature, and though the surveyors would " feel " that they lived in an Euclidean space they would discover their error sooner or later, depending on the amount of the curvature. The ancients thought that the world was flat and there is still an Act, dated 1870, on the Statute Book which forbids those who quote for the construction of railways and canals to make any allowance for " the alleged curvature of the earth " (129). Yet surveyors have been forced to allow for the curvature of the earth by the earth. In this century astronomers have been forced by their measurements to accept as a fact the negative curvature of the four-dimensional continuum which is their space. These sidelights are introduced to illustrate a point which can be proved mathematically, that the curvature of a manifold can be deduced from measurements made within that manifold without the advantage of a viewpoint involving a further dimension.

When considering Mercator charts we saw that some geodesics of the surface of the earth could be represented as straight lines on an Euclidean plane, though the majority cannot. Except for the difficulty that an infinitely long piece of paper is needed if we want to include the poles, all geodesics of the earth's surface can be mapped on such a chart by curved lines. In the same way, all the geodesics of visual space may be mapped in Euclidean space as curved lines and some as straight lines. This representation is easy to visualise and seems to be the most helpful.

Such then is Luneburg's theory of binocular vision, and it is, perhaps, necessary to repeat that as it is a mathematical theory; it is a unified description of a number of phenomena rather than an explanation of them. From observed facts Luneburg deduces the metric of the manifold in which these facts will, of necessity, be observed. It is not part of a mathematician's or a physicist's job to say why this is the metric of visual space, any more than why astronomic space should have a metric of the same form.

In describing Luneburg's theory I have used phenomena such as the horopters and the alley experiments to show the nature of the curvature of visual space. Luneburg derived the metric

$$ds^2 = \left(\frac{2}{e^{\sigma\gamma} + Ke^{-\sigma\gamma}}\right)^2 (\sigma^2 d\gamma^2 + d\phi^2 + \cos^2\phi d\theta^2)$$

where δ and K are individual constants, from more elementary premises by purely mathematical means, and as a check derived the form of the horopters and the alley from it. It seemed impossible to follow this development in non-mathematical language, so this simplified presentation has been adopted, but the reader should bear in mind that in the original the theory is on a sounder basis than it is here, in that it brings known facts, which were not used to deduce it, under one economical explanation.

One more phenomenon may be mentioned as a consequence of Luneburg's theory and that is our impression of the constancy of size. We have already noticed that though the retinal image is reduced in size as the object recedes from an observer, his impression of size remains very constant. This, moreover, remains true in the absence of other clues and at distances too large for the binocular parallax of the object to be significant, distances far too great for the observer's knowledge of his convergence to help. This constancy of size follows as a necessary corollary if the geometry of visual space is one of negative curvature but for no other geometry of constant curvature.

The metric given above may also be written in the form

$$ds^2 = \left(\frac{1}{\sinh^2\sigma(\gamma + \mu)}\right)(\sigma^2 d\gamma^2 + d\phi^2 + \cos^2\phi d\theta^2)$$

where σ and μ are the personal constants. This implies a scale of size which contracts for increasing values of γ proportionally to the expression $1/\sinh^2\sigma(\gamma + \mu)$. Luneburg suggested that there should be a physiological basis for so well defined a contraction, either in the eyes, the visual pathways, or in the cortex. I hope to show a possible basis later in this chapter.

It is a matter for the greatest regret that Luneburg's untimely death should have robbed the world of so original a mind, and at least postponed the experimental work which had been started on the basis of this theory.

From the chronological point of view, it would have been more logical to discuss Tschermak's conclusions on binocular vision before describing Luneburg's theory. It would also seem fairer to put Tschermak first as he had stated all the essentials of Luneburg's theory in the form of a list of requirements for any theory of visual space perception (*optischer Raumsinn*) some years before. However, he stopped short of the mathematical formulation of his conclusions. It appears unlikely that Luneburg knew of Tschermak's work at the time that he was working out his own theory, and as the writer is personally more indebted to Luneburg than to Tschermak, it seemed convenient to describe his work before proceeding to summarise Tschermak's conclusions. It will be seen that there is no conflict between them at any point.

In the section of the monumental *Handbuch der Physiologie* dealing with visual space perception, Tschermak lists eight fundamental facts which must be accounted for by any theory of binocular vision (131*a*). These eight fundamental facts, somewhat compressed, are:—

1. The fact of the appearance of visual impressions as outside our bodies in an egocentric organisation with respect to the meridional, horizontal, and frontal principal planes of the observer.
2. The fact that visual impressions lack a permanent constancy in the apparent directions of their components with respect to the observer.
3. The fact that the relative arrangement of the impressions do not correspond exactly with the relative geometrical positions of the stimuli.
4. The fact that the centre of rotation of the eye, the functional nodal point (which Tschermak calls the dioptric centre of perspective) and the centre about which retinal local signs are organised do not coincide.
5. The fact that subjective localisation with respect to defined retinal meridians is modified by such factors as the inclination of the head.
6. The fact that impressions from the two eyes are jointly referred to one common egocentric point.
7. The fact that cross-disparity between the impressions of the two eyes brings about a relative orientation with respect to depth, a binocular depth perception, and this without the intervention of ocular movement.
8. The fact that, under all normal conditions of binocular vision, objects at rest appear to be at rest and objects in motion appear to be in motion whether the observer is at rest or in motion, and whether he is moving his eyes or not.

Before proceeding to consider the conclusions that Tschermak draws, it is necessary to define his functional nodal point and the centre of organisation of local sign (131). The former he defines as the point where lines joining object points with their corresponding retinal image points intersect. Optically this should approximate to the posterior nodal point. Tschermak quotes 7·4 mm. behind the corneal vertex for axial objects, and as much as 8·9 mm. behind it for highly oblique rays. Experiments with chess board patterns show that patterns subtending equal angles at the nodal point do not appear square and rectilinear. He states that there is a centre about which equal arcs of the retina do correspond to equal directional intervals in space when projected outwards from the nodal point; this centre appears to lie some 4 mm. in front of the posterior nodal point and close to the entrance pupil of the eye.*

Tschermak then points out that theories of space perception fall under three main headings, though some theories may combine elements from two, or all three of them. These three headings are:—

I. *Projection Theories.* Theories where the sensation is located at the intersection of two lines drawn on optical principles.

II. *Local Sign Theories*, which embrace those theories which assume special properties for individual retinal elements.

III. *Oculo-Motor Theories.* Those theories which make our sense location in space depend either on proprioception from the extraocular muscles, or from knowledge of the intended movement of the eyes.

Projection theories are the most obvious and the most economical of hypotheses, and it is natural that they should have been embraced by the earlier workers. Volkmann (139), Nagel, Donders, and to some extent Helmholtz, held that the eyes project their visual impressions outward into space and von Kreis, in an appendix to the third volume of Helmholtz, proposes a bicentric projection, which is the forerunner of a theory that has been advanced lately and which, in some measure, anticipates Luneburg's bipolar co-ordinate handling of the subject, though the latter theory is not a projection theory.

It is obvious that no projection theory can account for the first three of Tschermak's facts, and that it is difficult to explain No. 6, the fact that we project from a binoculus, unless the theory be complicated to an intolerable degree; one feels a certain sympathy with a recent speculator who prefers to deny the existence of a binoculus. The insuperable difficulty for any projection theory is the lack of identity between subjective and objective location and the fact that such theories, even when their advocates pay the fullest lip service to the psychological aspects of the problem, leave no room for psychology to play its part in space perception.

The solution of this difficulty, and most other difficulties, lies in " the theory of retinal local signs, or functional space values ", originated by Lotze (95) and extended by Hering, Stumf, and others, including Tschermak himself, thus reconciling the purely psychological with the psycho-physiological aspects of the problem. Here to each individual element of the visual organ, which must be taken to include the retina,

* It, therefore, also lies very close to the surface of the retinal sphere if it were continued. From such a centre equal arcs would, geometrically, subtend equal angles.

visual pathways and cortex, a functional quality, or height and breadth value, is ascribed (and, on concerted action, a depth value) as a primary independent attribute. This function being, in principle, independent of lines of sight and, indeed, independent even of the position of the element within the retinal mosaic. Visual location depends, according to this view, in the first place, on the independent local sign or space value of the individual mosaic element of the visual organ. However, the visual direction (as well as the subjective distance of observation) is not permanently settled as such, rather is it given only in the form of an ordering, while the size value is given by the prevailing scale of height, breadth and depth; the local signs represent functional arrangement values, not constant functional size values.

It is obvious that the whole of this follows from Luneburg's contention that we have no direct knowledge of the angles ϕ, θ, and γ in his treatment, but only of $d\phi$, $d\theta$ and $d\gamma$. In view of the finite structure of the retina and the limited number of fibres connecting it with the cortex, the writer considers that $\delta\phi$, $\delta\theta$ and $\delta\gamma$ represent what we appreciate more correctly.

In binocular vision Tschermak postulates in contra-distinction to the bicentric projection theory, a paired agreement in local sign, a common visual direction, without the assumption of a complete identity of corresponding points. He attributes the apparent stability of the scene when the subject moves or inclines his head, as indeed do most theories, to the modifying effects of muscle proprioception, labyrinthine stimuli and knowledge of ocular movements conveyed to the higher centres.

Oculo-motor or myogenic theories, such as those of Steinbach, Wundt (159), and Cornelius, among others, attribute visual localisation to knowledge of the fixation movements of the eye, whether this is obtained from kinæsthetic sources, as many authors have suggested (this view has gained support from the recent researches of Cooper and Daniel (41)) or from innervation sensation or " felt will " as originally suggested by Meynert and Helmholtz. Tschermak considered that the organisation of local sign about a centre well in advance of the centre of rotation was of itself a conclusive proof that space perception did not depend on muscle sense, though he seems to have thought it possible that it may have an influence in providing the size scale of visual space.

If we accept a theory of space perception based on retinal local signs, and it seems impossible not to do so, we are immediately faced with the question: Are these local signs innate or learned by experience? This question has divided students of the psychology of vision into two camps from the earliest days of the science. Even before the subject could be said to have become differentiated, philosophers were divided into opposing schools of thought on the question of whether our conception of physical space is innate or acquired; Kant, in his " Critic of Pure Reason " (1787) having, according to Duke-Elder, been the leader of what has become the Nativistic School, while Locke, a century earlier, in the " Essay Concerning Human Understanding " (1690), held the contrary view and may be considered to be the founder of the Empirical School.

Naturally Lotze, as the originator of the theory of local signs, belonged to the nativistic school, as did Panum (110), Hering, Tschermak, Verhoeff, and Luneburg, though the views held by the last three allow scope for the influence of experience on the final percept. On the other side, Nagel and Wundt were among the first to make a comprehensive attempt to develop a theory of space perception on empiristic grounds, while the giant figure in that camp is, of course, Helmholtz. Duke-Elder (49) holds the balance so true in recording the pioneer work on the subject that it is almost impossible to judge his own views. It seems likely that he tends, as does the writer, to accept a nativistic basis which can be modified by experience.

The arguments that Tschermak advanced for the nativistic basis of local signs are that the congenitally blind locate pressure phosphenes as normal individuals do; the localising ability of new-born animals; the defined anatomical relationship between areas of the visual cortex and the visual fields, as shown by cortical injuries. The possibility of abnormal retinal correspondence has been advanced as evidence for the empiristic view, but as Tschermak points out, such correspondences are never so static or so fully developed as a normal correspondence. The fact that patients with abnormal retinal correspondence sometimes experience monocular diplopia during the process of cure seems to me to prove that the true correspondence has not been changed but has been inhibited while a new correspondence was acquired. In the writer's experience, once the inhibition of the normal correspondence has been overcome it is immediately manifested in its full development and does not require training. One of the most convincing proofs of the fixity of correspondence is that aniseikonia can be demonstrated, both in those with symptoms and those without, with remarkable consistency, whereas if local signs had an empirical basis the subject would not only adapt himself to the condition from a subjective point of view but would reorganise his local sign correspondence so that the condition would cease to be demonstrable.

It seems then that we must accept a nativistic origin for retinal local signs so far as direction is concerned, the next question is: Has our stereoscopic sense of depth a nativistic a basis? Again, the author finds himself in agreement with Tschermak who holds that an appreciation of the significance of cross disparities (*Querdifferenz*) of the two images is innate so far as the determination of order (*Ordung*) is concerned, but that factors of size and scale have to be learned from experience. This is equivalent to Luneburg's view that we have direct appreciation of $d\gamma$, or of $\delta\gamma$, but that the constant of integration must be supplied by experience. On this view the story of Helmholtz, as a small boy, asking his mother to reach him down one of the statues on a tower in Potsdam, which he had taken for a doll just out of his own reach, no longer conflicts with a nativistic view of local sign.

Verhoeff (136) in " A New Theory of Binocular Vision ", which we shall discuss shortly, also takes a nativistic view both for " unification ", a process which he substitutes for fusion, and for perception of depth. He makes the reservation, which is in conformity with the views given above, that experience may be necessary to enable consciousness to evaluate the information passed to it. As a reason for rejecting the empiristic view he cites a case of his own (138) of abnormal correspondence where the angle of anomaly for distant vision differed by more than five degrees from that for near vision.

In justice to the empiristic school, it is necessary to point out that differences of correspondence between distant and near vision can be demonstrated in normal individuals by means of the retinal slip experiments described in the last chapter. These differences are, however, of a quite different order and are the result of the flexibility of correspondence necessary for the simultaneous single vision of two object points allowed by Panum's fusion areas.

Verhoeff claims that while the two retinal images are represented separately and simultaneously somewhere in the brain, only one of the two representations of any pair of corresponding retinal units can be present in consciousness at any given moment, the conscious image being built up of elements from the two uniocular images. It may consist entirely of elements from one eye or the other, or it may be compounded from the two, with the stipulation that the representation of one or other of two corresponding points must always disappear from consciousness. In particular, the points of occlusion in the monocular view being replaced by background points from the other image, the term replacement being substituted for suppression.

Verhoeff rejects the conception of fusion as understood by most other writers, namely as a process whereby one unit of a sensation is produced by combining two units of stimulus. In its place he postulates a mechanism of " unification ", which appears to imply the construction of a single mental concept by a process of selecting point by point that one of the two corresponding unit stimuli which will best serve the mind's immediate purpose. He describes the process whereby two images appear to fuse and give stereopsis as quasi-unification, still contending that one has disappeared, and asserts that when one of a pair of disparate images disappears during stereopsis the position of its fellow remains unchanged. The reason for the use of the term quasi-unification here, instead of unification, appears to be that it is sometimes possible to get a sense of depth from objects seen in physiological diplopia. He observes that it is possible for an invisible image to affect a visible one, presumably in the sense of depth conveyed.

This theory closely resembles that of Cantonnet (25), who held that stereoscopic vision results from the selective suppression of elements from two views of the object seen in physiological diplopia.

A further theory which must be mentioned is that of Hering which is illustrated by Figure VI, 1, reproduced from Hartridge (68). It will be seen that, according to this theory, stereoscopy is the result of one retinal element of one eye being brought into correspondence with two or more of the other. This theory has been revived lately in the form of saying that one eye defines the line of sight while the other measures off the intercepts upon it. The present writer has shown (28) that when the conditions of the figure are fulfilled the observer gets no sense of depth from the farther object point. It is also difficult to see how Hering reconciled this theory with his belief in nativistic local signs.

In the form in which Elliman has tried to revive this theory he has contrived to wed to it Verhoeff's points of monocular occlusion on the background. In the writer's view, it is impossible to assign to them any functional rôle in stereoscopic vision. They are not even available to inspection by introspection, or any method such as those by which one can demonstrate the blind spot. The only way of demonstrating them that I know is the demonstration, alluded to above, that we have no stereoscopic sense of depth on points visible to one eye only.

These points of occlusion are self-sealing, as is the blind spot, in that the only interruption of the background that enters consciousness is the binocular point of occlusion. The mechanism of this sealing must be that which Verhoeff describes as replacement, with this important reservation, that it is possible to mark the two points of monocular occlusion on a background so that each of these marks is visible to one eye only, and, in binocular vision, see both marks with the occluding target apparently covering a point of binocular occlusion between them, at the same time that a third witness point, on the background, is seen singly. The " repair " of images is discussed very fully by Hartridge (67).

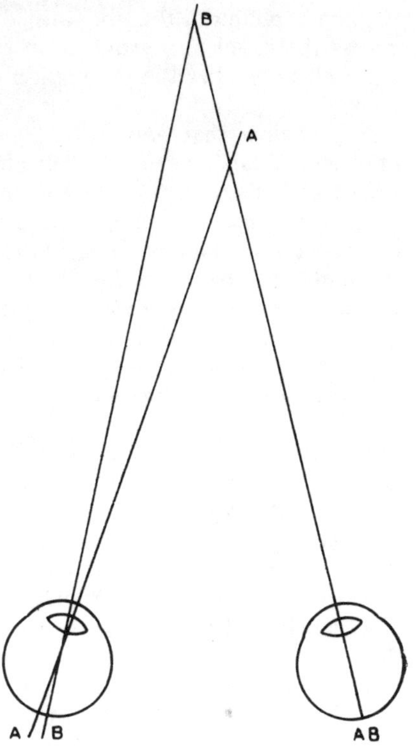

FIG. VI 1.

The writer finds it impossible to agree with Verhoeff in rejecting the conception of true fusion where two disparate elements from the images from the two eyes are combined to form one sensation presented to consciousness which differs from both those which go to form it. We saw from experiments with the stereogram reproduced as Fig. IV, 11, that the addition of a marker gap to Verhoeff's figure shows that the central line in the circle has not been replaced, but has been fused with one or other of the two lines in the other half of the stereogram, and that it is this fused line alone which stands out either behind or in front of the figure. We also saw from Fig. IV, 12, how different observers could fuse the same figures in different ways and each get the impression that he expected from it.

We know that our subconscious knowledge of convergence plays a part in our estimates of both distance and size. If two targets are fused by over-convergence and then separated, not only does the resulting fused image appear to come nearer as convergence increases, but it also appears to become smaller; the reverse effect can be caused by diverging. It is interesting to note that this is an effect which becomes less and less easy to observe as we practise it. Long practise at diverging his eyes for fusing stereograms has completely robbed the writer of the power of making a phantom thumb, formed by fusing his own two thumbs, travel across the room and grow to an enormous size as it does so, though he can well remember the impression of that occurring in his earliest experiments.

It is clear that only muscle sense or knowledge of the intended eye movements can give us any absolute measure of distance, or supply us with a scale factor or constant of integration which will make our location of external objects anything more than relative in situations where experience or expectation does not provide the key. Yet we also know how easily the mind sets aside the data from convergence from the fact that stereoscopic range finders always see the reference mark move and not the target, so long as there is any target in the binocular field of view which the mind can think of as relatively fixed.

We noticed in an earlier chapter that the introduction of prisms, to allow the eyes to turn so as to project the fused image in the appropriate direction, relieved the discomfort caused by fusing two circles of different sizes. This tends to show that the mind makes use of overall size disparities in assessing the direction in which objects lie; it also provides a possible explanation for the so-called " induced size effect ", whereby a meridional size lens giving magnification in the vertical meridian causes the same spatial disorientation as a similar lens, though of less power, placed before the other eye so as to magnify in the horizontal meridian, the suggestion being that the vertical magnification, which has no meaning, is resolved into an overall magnification to one eye, with a directional significance and a horizontal magnification to the other eye which rotates the frontal plane about a vertical axis.

Under rigidly controlled conditions, monocular vision gives no sense of depth, but under normal conditions there are so many clues from the " context " that the scene appears almost as solid to one-eyed vision as to two-eyed vision. It is true that those who are accustomed to good binocular vision miss it if they are suddenly deprived of it, as the writer can testify from his experience of experiments on monocular occlusion. But, as we have seen, when there is conflict between the evidence of monocular vision and that from purely binocular vision, monocular vision almost always wins, and when it does not win, the mind generally makes some concession to it, such as a hole in the wall to allow the lamp post, seen pseudoscopically, to get to its anomalous position.

This overriding authority which monocular clues seem to possess over binocular evidence is not surprising when we remember that, on the theory of space perception elaborated by Tschermak from the work of Lotze, Hering, and others, and formulated by Luneburg, binocular vision requires some outside factor to give it scale. This outside factor has to be capable of enforcing the choice by the mind of one out of an infinity of possible solutions. The mind's insistence on the rectangular solution, even when the objective stimulus is a distorted room congruent to a given rectangular room, is a good illustration of the power of this scale factor. In the author's view, the personal constants in Luneburg's metric for visual space and the arbitrary constants of integration that such an equation implies leave all the room necessary for the most generous allowance for psychological factors without there being any need to elaborate theories which depend on introspection and deny the evidence of experiment.

Cantonnet's contention that stereoscopy is the result of the selective suppression of elements from two views seen in physiological diplopia takes no account of the fact that physiological diplopia can be of two forms: the true physiological, or the introspection diplopia where, normally, one image is ignored but can be recalled to consciousness without affecting the position occupied by the image already perceived. On the other hand, when viewing the small targets whose difference in distance places them fairly close to the limit of simultaneous single binocular vision, it is easy to an experienced observer to break fusion on either, while holding it on the other, and to watch the two diplopic images approaching and receding from each other as the disparity is reduced. This becomes more and more difficult until finally it becomes impossible. While it is true that some sense of depth is possible with unfused images seen in physiological diplopia, the elimination of one diplopic image, as opposed to its fusion with its fellow, destroys all sense of depth in every experiment of which the writer knows.

Considerations affecting monocular visual acuity do not strictly fall within the limits set by the title of this essay, but they are so important to our subject that it would be wrong to pass them by without a mention. The ability of the eye to detect a break in the alignment of two lines far smaller than a cone unit in angle has long been known, and its explanation has been the subject of much discussion. The eye is also able to detect differences corresponding to far less than a cone unit in size between adjacent objects. Hering suggested that the explanation was that the eye performed constant small scanning movements which enabled the brain to assess finer detail by some averaging process. This theory has been supported recently by Wright (158). The fact that Lord and Wright record larger involuntary eye movements with a subject in the prone position than Hartridge and Thomson (69) do in the erect, when taken in conjunction with the writer's observation (33) that visual acuity is substantially less in the prone position than in the erect position, seems to go far to disprove this theory.

It has been shown by Hecht and Mintz, Shlaer, and others (68) that a difference in illumination between one cone and its neighbours of as little as two per cent, or even less, can, under suitable conditions, be appreciated; a single black line being detectable, under optimum conditions, when the illumination of the darkest part of its retinal image was only 0·5 to 1 per cent below that of the background. The writer agrees with Hartridge that this implies some form of central repair of the image analogous to the anti-chromatic responses which eliminate colour fringes. The fact that binocular acuity is generally somewhat higher than monocular strongly supports this idea. That the blind spot is never present in consciousness, even in monocular vision, shows the mind's ability to effect repairs.

The author agrees with Tschermak that his list of requirements is best met by a theory based on retinal local signs of nativistic origin, not only for up and down and right and left, but also in depth, with the reservation that these do not give absolute geometrical localisations in space. Speaking particularly of the sense of depth to be derived from retinal disparities, Tschermak held this to be innate but only to place points in order. This is half of Luneburg's requirement for mathematical treatment, and if the ordering be conceded the comparison of differences will also be conceded. This conception of Tschermak's seems to have been made in common with Cayley's and Silvester's conception of mathematical invariance.

Luneburg's mathematical analysis seems to describe all the known facts of binocular space perception in a most economical manner. It is a theory in the mathematical sense, though from the physiological point of view it is, as has already been said, a description, but it is a most suggestive description in that it defines more clearly than anything that has gone before the precise nature of the problems, in the mathematical sense, that the central mechanism has to solve, and so offers a starting point for speculation about the possible nature of that mechanism.

It seems clear that the central problem of binocular vision is that of solving the differential equation quoted above. Such equations generally possess an infinite family of solutions, though only one can be present in consciousness at any given moment. Certain well known inadequate representations, such as Schroeder's staircase, or the pattern shown in Figure VI, 2, are capable of two solutions which are acceptable to the mind, and the question of which presents itself at any moment, particularly in the case of the figure given here, seems to be a matter of pure chance. Generally speaking, the solution presented to the mind will be uniquely determined by some factor supplied from experience which does not strictly belong to binocular vision. Furthermore, the monocular clues may be sufficient, by themselves, to enable the mind to construct a three-dimensional concept, and it may be, as in pseudoscopic vision, that that concept is not compatible with the differential equation of binocular vision. When this occurs, one or other solution has to be rejected; this may occur in whole or in part. It seems probable that when monocular vision and binocular vision are incompatible the concept presented to consciousness is made up partly from the one and partly from the other.

We may say that the human binocular apparatus consists of two eyes whose retinæ are endowed with local signs for Luneburg's $\delta\theta$ and $\delta\phi$ and whose cross disparities possess the property of providing the local signs for $\delta\gamma$. The retinæ of these two eyes are connected point for point so as to conserve their local signs to the occipital cortex, which functions as a computing mechanism which evaluates the equations defined by the metric of visual space, but which requires to be supplied with a constant of integration, at least, before it can produce a unique solution. This constant is supplied presumably by the visual association areas and is capable of enforcing a solution very different from the physical stimulus, as we have seen in the case of the congruent rooms. In that central mechanism, a single representation is built up which, in general, differs from each of the monocular representations, not as suggested by Cantonnet and Verhoeff by being built up of elements from each, but by being built up of new elements to the making of each of which each uniocular image has contributed.

In his Lister Oration to the Royal College of Surgeons, Professor Jefferson (76) warned the medical profession against the danger of trying

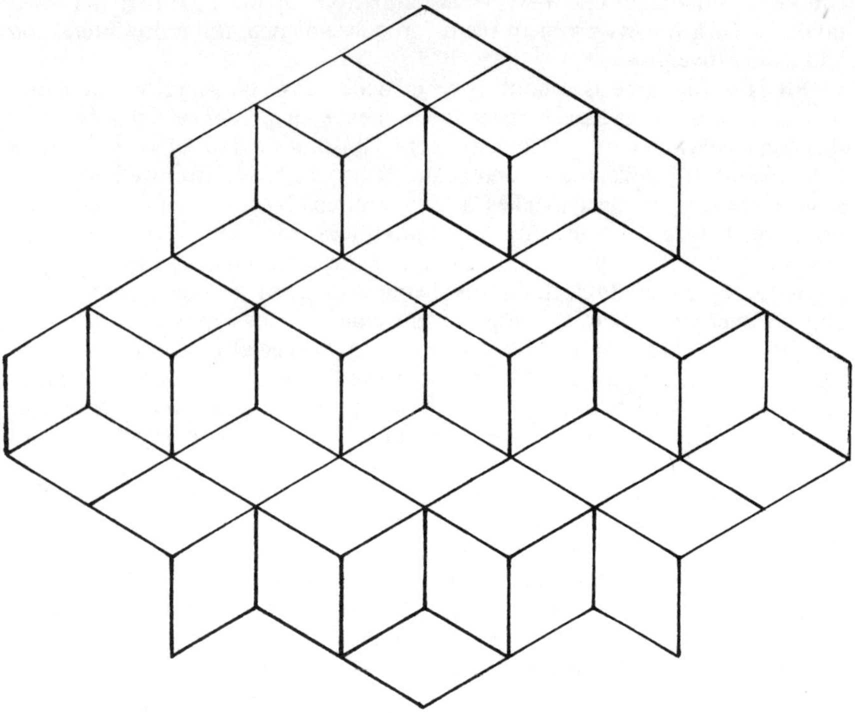

Fig. VI. 2.

to push the analogy between electronic computing machines and the brain too far. However, he was especially concerned in insisting on the essential difference between brain and mind, urging his hearers to remember that while the analogue might be helpful in the study of the cortex, the machine had no mind, as we understand the term. He says: " Discussion of mind-brain relations is, I know well, premature, but I suspect that it always will be premature ". This is a view with which the author humbly agrees, but as one of the first, in this country, to attempt to illustrate the working of the occipital cortex by analogy with electronic computers (35), he still feels that the possible utility of the analogy is by no means exhausted.

It seems probable to the author that the solution of Luneburg's equation is effected in the occipital cortex with considerable and almost constant speed, and that it is this mechanism which is operating, almost alone in most of the controlled experiments on disparity stereopsis that we have considered. It is true that we may take some time in making our final judgment when the retinal disparities are near the limit of resolution, but that may well be due to our making several assessments and then comparing them. The writer's own introspective impression favours this hypothesis but it must not be regarded as evidence. There is no doubt that normally our sense of depth operates very quickly, and that where no confusion can arise the variations in its speed of operation are not large enough to enter consciousness. The fact that on occasion stereoscopy can be so slow a process that we are conscious of the time that the mind takes to work out its problem seems, in consequence, the more interesting and suggestive.

It is when there is a conflict of evidence and the mind has difficulty in reconciling the evidence from disparities with preconceived ideas that this long delay occurs. If one suddenly puts on a pair of size lenses in a room full of intellectually significant detail, such as furniture and right-angled corners, it always takes a very appreciable time, often a minute or more, before the full sensation that things have changed their shape develops. Some subjects even fail to see the effect at all in a room, the influence of psychological factors being too great for stereopsis to be able to overcome them. These context clues, as they may be called, are far less potent in unfamiliar surroundings, especially where binocular clues abound, such as a leaf room, but even here the changes take place far more slowly than the build up and collapse of the sense of depth that one experiences when the second view of a pair of stereograms is exposed or concealed.

The conclusion which forces itself on the writer's mind is that this latter time represents the time taken to solve Luneburg's equation and for consciousness to sanction the solution in a simple case where no conflict arises. The extreme times for solution seem to imply that the final percept is the result of repeated, subconscious " trial and error " matching, the mind making further and further concessions to visual evidence until a stable percept is present in consciousness. Alternatively, the mind may reject the purely binocular evidence and accept only that from previous experience or other evidence.

It will be seen that this hypothesis, while attempting to illustrate one stage of binocular vision, allows all the necessary freedoms for the effects of psychological factors. In the writer's opinion, acceptance of these views reduces many of the phenomena to which psychologists have attached importance to somewhat ignominious position of being " just what one would expect ". The fact that we see a foreshortened circle as a circle and not as an ellipse is to be expected if there is a mechanism for applying scale factors from experience to supply the necessary constants of integration. If such a mechanism will work with binocular vision, how much more easily will it not work with monocular vision? Another instance of a phenomenon to which psychologists have attached importance but which now seems trivial is that provided part of a figure is seen binocularly, in a stereopair, portions which are continuous with that part will be referred to the same distance, such as the fork with the handle on one half of the card and the prongs on the other, cited by Professor Bartlett (13).

The scale or correction factors clearly depend on memory for their operation and so, on experience, to that extent the author is in complete agreement with the Gestalt School, but he is also in agreement with Professor Jefferson that the brain-mind relationship is out of reach. It may be possible, in the near future, to speculate on the cortical mechanism of memory and such speculations may prove fruitful. Many calculating machines have memories both for numbers and for instructions, some of the static mechanised model type, the more modern ones being generally of the type where impulses circulate continuously in a closed system. The present writer, at all events, is not qualified to pursue this analogy further.

When we turn to the visual cortex proper, the position is somewhat different. Its relative isolation from the rest of the brain facilitates its study and seems to justify an attempt to illustrate possible methods by which it might function. The basic requirement for making a computing machine is a mechanism where if two impulses are fed in one comes out. It is obvious that a sufficient number of such units would enable one to construct an adding machine, operating in the binary scale, of any capacity desired, and the repeated operations of addition and subtraction (which is the equivalent of the addition of the complement) will suffice for the performance of all the operations of arithmetic, including the process of integration from finite differences. We shall see however that, granted a two-in-one-out mechanism, a far simpler scheme than numerical integration can be suggested as the modus operandi of the visual cortex.

It becomes necessary to enquire whether there is any evidence for the existence of a two-in-one-out arrangement in other parts of the central nervous system. Van der Velden (134) found that two quanta of light acting on the visual purple of two cones were the minimum that could be appreciated as a flash of light. Other workers have given different results, but some of the earliest even were very close to this figure. Throughout the central nervous system we have the phenomenon of facilitation and inhibition, so it does not seem to the writer that there is need to go further in justifying the tentative assumption that some mechanism of a two-in-one-out nature may exist in the cortex.

There are many possible computing layouts which could solve the problems that we are considering. The considerations which govern our choice are economy of means and compatibility with what we know of the histology and physiology of the cortex. But even if we were to ignore the histology of the cortex, the chances are that we would choose a layout of interconnected cells in which the active cells formed an approximate representation of the external scene which provided the physical stimulus as the most economical arrangement.

The words "approximate representation" are important as we have in the cortex a one-to-one representation of the retinæ spread over an elaborate surface. This representation is highly distorted, the macular area is represented by an extent of cortical surface which is vastly in excess of its topographical importance. Since the macular area includes the object of attention at any moment, its representation as an area of cortex appears to be approximately proportional to its interest.

That portion of the cortex whose surface represents an approximate map of our visual field possesses depth as well as surface, and so is capable of providing a conformal representation of a three-dimensional scene. Granted a point to point representation of two dimensions of the external scene over the surface of the cortex, and the evidence for that is conclusive, if the cortex itself has depth, a three-dimensional representation is an obvious possibility. Such a representation cannot properly be described as a model but it may, none the less, be a faithful point for point representation of the scene which is the stimulus for it. A representation in depth of a point in front of the plane of the horopter and behind it, spread over the convolutions of the cortex may not at first sight have much in common with a model of the physical stimulus, yet it can easily be seen that it may conform rigidly with the rules of mathematical invariance. This is no more than saying that, for all purposes of visualising its function, the cortex may be regarded as spread out over a flat surface and submitted to any elastic deformation which will cause it to represent the frontal plane.

We must now recall the histology of the visual cortex. The outstanding difference between it and other areas is the so-called white line or stria of Gennari. This is so well marked that it is visible in sections to the naked eye and so gives to this region the name " area striata ". It seems clearly established that this white line of Gennari which splits up layer IV of the visual cortex and which is found nowhere else is the cortical projection of the optic radiations. These are the oblique fibre bundles seen in sections of the cortex which undergo degeneration if the optic radiations are cut, but which survive isolation from the rest of the cortex. Le Gros Clark (84) found that these fibres terminate in layer IV and in the outer granular layer II. Polyak has suggested (113*a*) and Le Gros Clark and Sunderland (92) have confirmed by degeneration experiments that the radial bundles, which are a familiar feature of all representations of the visual cortex, are association fibres from immediately adjacent areas. No such fibres have ever been traced for more than a very few millimetres.

A possible layout has been devised for an electronic gear devised to enable the blind to read normal print from sounds produced by scanning the page with a photoelectric device. Wiener (145) records that von Bonin, the neurophysiologist, mistook a diagram of that instrument for a schema of the occipital cortex. Fig. VI, 3, is a possible schema for a stereo vision computer; a similar error would be possible here. Input lines (or fibres if we push the analogy and attempt to apply it to the cortex) from one source are shown solid while those from the other are dotted. Eight of them, drawn heavier, are carrying signals in pairs as indicated by the brackets. In one pair there is no disparity, the remaining three show disparities varying in amount and sign. The circles represent quiescent electronic units, while those which have been excited by receiving paired impulses are shown filled in; possible interconnection channels are shown broken, while those in use at the moment are completed.

The requirements for such a system to operate are two in number, the two-in-one-out condition which we have already examined, and secondly some arrangement for keeping the signals in pairs. It will be seen from the figure that if the two pairs of signals on the right change partners, the two units indicated as stars will be activated instead of those shown black, and in one case the alternative unit is the nearest to a possible input pair. However, the diagram is very much condensed; if the organisation of the visual cortex should prove to be on comparable lines it must certainly possess far more interconnections, and the big changes in disparity which we see in the diagram would not occur. In electronic engineering some form of time gating would be the simplest way to guard against such a result, signals being sent off in pairs at intervals.

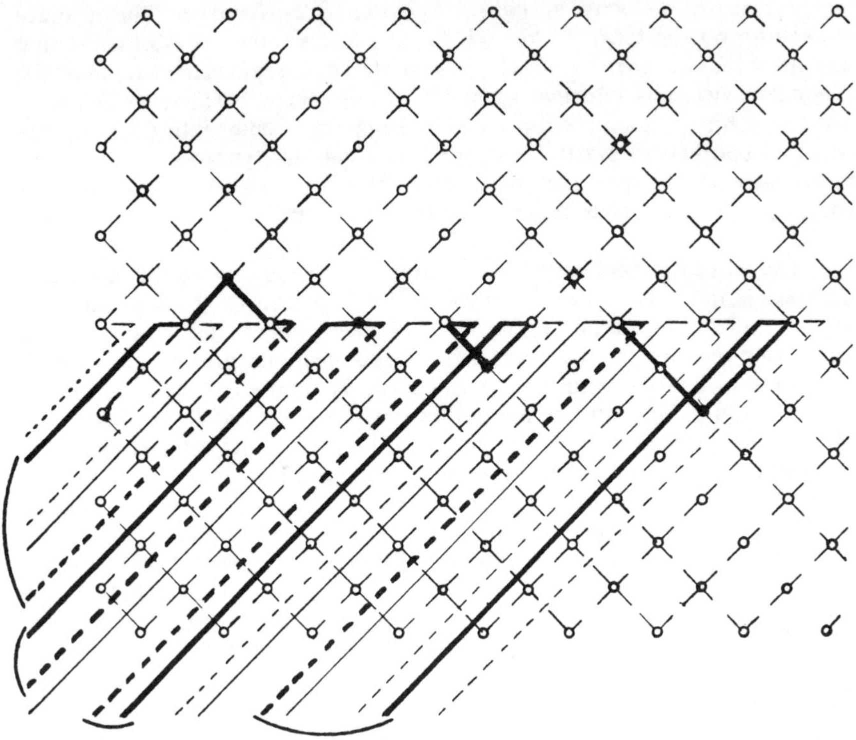

Fig. VI. 3.

It seems probable that no such precautions would be necessary in the cortex. Except at discontinuities where parts of the scene will only be seen monocularly, changes of disparity occur gradually and an arrangement which allowed the first possible unit to receive its double impulse would be adequate, provided that the active unit blocked all patterns that passed through it. Sherrington's work indicates that such a provision is to be found everywhere in the central nervous system.

It will be noticed that we have tacitly assumed, in order to define the sign of the disparities, that impulses from one input system are propagated solely along one set of diagonals, while those from the other input system are propagated at right angles to them. This would not be difficult to arrange electronically; whether any comparable phenomenon occurs anywhere in the central nervous system is beyond the writer's knowledge. However, other methods of achieving the same result are possible.

The writer does not want to push the analogy much further. It has been developed to this point because it may indicate a possible physiological basis, such as Luneburg felt to be necessary, for the hyperbolic metric of subject space. As we saw above, our scale of size is, according to Luneburg, proportional to $1/\sinh \sigma (\gamma + \mu)$ which implies that it contracts with increasing values of γ. The space time continuum of relativity also has a hyperbolic metric developed from the general line element

$$ds^2 = dx^2 + dy^2 + dz^2 - c^2dt^2$$

where c is the velocity of light. The departure from Euclidean space depending on the term $-c^2dt^2$ which introduces time. It is obvious that any effect that the term $-c^2dt^2$ can have in the small regions of space in which binocular vision is effective must be utterly negligible; nevertheless, it gives us a hint to look for a place where time does enter into the workings of our hypothetical system, and we find it at the synapses. Some time is lost at each synapse and the greater the disparities, the more synapses the impulses must pass before meeting at the cell that they can jointly excite.

The difficulty that leaps to the mind when looking at the schematic diagram is that such an arrangement cannot account for such phenomena as the Pulfrich effect or the Verhoeff-Fincham effect, but that is due to over simplification; only four possible connections are shown to each unit in the diagram and the arrangement is limited to rigid rectilinear transmission. The cells in the cortex are not arranged in straight lines, nor are they limited to four dendrites. If, as appears probable, a reduction in illumination involves an increase in the time lost at the synapses, or as Bannister (9) suggests, in an increase in retinal action time, or both, the conditions necessary for both phenomena are fulfilled.

The study of cerebral rhythm and of the wave forms of visual impulses when they reach the cortex has not reached a stage where it helps us to understand how the cortex unites the two uniocular images. Adrian and Matthews (3*a*) have demonstrated two electrical ryhthms, one of which appears to be connected with vision, or at least affected by visual stimuli. This is known as the alpha rhythm, with a normal frequency of about 10 cycles per second, but capable of following the frequency of a flickering light stimulus between about eight and twenty cycles per second. This seems too slow and too irregular to perform the functions of a synchronizing or gating pulse, and, moreover, is most in evidence when the eyes are shut or when gazing at a blank wall; any attempt to see appears to destroy it. The beta rhythm has a frequency of between 20 and 40 per second, and so might have served our purpose were it not that it seems to arise principally in more anterior portions of the cortex and to respond to tactile stimuli rather than light. At present, it seems that we must look to a wave form with a sharp rise, preferably to a spike rather than to a gating rhythm, if we feel the need for a factor to bring the two input impulses together at one receptor unit.

On any basis such as we have been considering monocular vision and diplopia require that an impulse shall be able to put some cell into a receptive state in which a second one along the same channel will trigger it into activity, or as an alternative, that the last cell to which the impulse travels, if it has failed to connect en route with its paired impulse, shall be able to respond to a single impulse. These cells would clearly not be part of the systems which built up the stereoscopic picture, but cells with no depth, or " any depth " significance.

Accepting these speculations for the moment, it seems impossible that any of these cells, the stereoscopic array and the " any depth " cells, can be the final conscious cells. There must be at least one more array whose activity is a compromise between the first set, which we have charged with the duty of setting up a geometrical representation, and the memory clues from the association areas. There are plenty of cells available; these might well be the final conscious cells.

It is important to repeat that all this is speculation about what might be and not a description of what is. The main purpose of this speculative description of a possible cortex is to illustrate the functions which the cortex must perform by attempting to follow them through a mechanism which could perform them. Although the author has tried to construct his mechanical cortex so as to resemble the histological cortex and is rather in love with the result, he has not forgotten that it is only a parable —a work of fiction. Two years ago, in the paper in which he first mentioned the possible analogy, he drew up his own list of facts which any theory of binocular vision must explain. Although some of his views have naturally changed in the meantime as the result of reading and experiment, this list still seems to him worth reproducing. They are the facts that:—

(*a*) Points other than the point of fixation will also be seen in single binocular vision, provided that their retinal disparity is not too great.

(*b*) If this disparity is too great to allow simultaneous fusion, physiological diplopia will occur unless the image formed by one eye, usually the non-dominant one, is suppressed.

(*c*) If the disparity is near the limit for simultaneous fusion, and if the pattern aids observation, the images seen in physiological diplopia may be seen gliding into fusion and out again. When this happens, both images normally move towards a mean position.

(*d*) The fusion of disparate images is more difficult if the disparity is such as to contradict other clues.

(*e*) The mind has no knowledge of the absolute value of the parallax angle of a given object, only of the difference between parallax angles.

(*f*) The mind can ignore stereopsis without suppressing the image of either eye; and will do so when stereopsis runs counter to its preconceived convictions.

(*g*) The suppression of stereopsis may cause discomfort.

(*h*) The mind is capable of seeing things which it has postulated in order to reconcile conflicting pieces of information.

(*i*) The mind utilises every component of image disparity, an overall size difference being a factor in our sense of direction.

(*j*) In some situations the mind has a choice of interpretation which it can place on the data available to it.

(*k*) When this occurs, the mind will generally choose the interpretation that fits in best with the other evidence available to it, from the present or the past. In some situations it can change from one interpretation to the other at will.

Although the writer would now re-word several of these " facts ", he still considers that they are all correct, and so has reproduced them as they were originally written. It is clear that there is nothing really new in his views on binocular vision, and certainly nothing that could be described as a new theory. However, they are more detailed and rather more comprehensive than any account that he knows, so it seems worth while to finish this monograph with a recapitulation of his conclusions. He believes that:—

The receptive elements of the two retinæ are endowed with local signs for direction, up and down, and right and left, and that disparities between the two retinæ order points in depth. These local signs of direction and this ordering in depth are innate, but they are not appreciated as actual magnitudes but as the result of summing small finite differences approximating to infinitesimal derivatives. As a consequence of this disparity stereopsis has no scale and is capable of many interpretations, the choice of interpretation being made in response to some outside factor. The most important of these is recollection of past experience which is generally able to select the scale factor which makes a solution compatible with the subject's expectations possible. In the absence of any other determining factor the mind's knowledge of the convergence of the eyes may supply a scale factor.

While the writer has always held that our knowledge of convergence played a part in the educating of disparity stereopsis, he held until fairly recently that an appreciation of depth from retinal disparities was acquired. He has now changed his views on this point and believes it to be nativistic. It is worth while noting that such a nativistic view explains why an infant can grasp something within reach as soon as it can control its binocular fixation, as this only requires making the two disparities equal and generally equal to zero, and yet the infant may still reach out for something well beyond its reach, as it has not enough experience to supply a scale factor and can discover that it cannot equalize the two disparities only by trying and failing.

The writer is still of the opinion that we have little or no true proprioception from the extraocular muscles, and that any knowledge that the mind has of convergence is the result of the order to converge being reported back, rather than the outcome being reported back. He does believe that the extraocular muscles play a most important and essential part in binocular vision and agrees with Wright (157) that the scanning of the scene in a manner which may be described as visual palpation allows the two foveæ to search the scene so that the mind may have the benefit of foveal acuity all over the surface of an object in integrating the changing retinal disparities. He does not, however, agree with those who would give any more important rôle to changes of convergence than is implied above.

Finally, the writer would repeat once again that, in his belief, we have no direct knowledge of the absolute values of direction, either in the lateral or vertical direction, or of the angle of convergence, and that they are appreciated only by a process of mathematical integration from differences.

REFERENCES

** These references have not been checked.*

1 Adamson, J., and Fincham, E. F.: *Trans. Ophth. Soc.*, LIX part I.

2 Adler, F. H.: *Arch. Ophth.*, XXXIII, 362.

3 Adrian, E. D., and Matthews, B. H. C.: *Brain*, LVII, 355.

3*a* Adrian, E. D., and Matthews, B. H. C.: *Brain*, LVIII, 323.

4 Ames, A., Jr., and Gliddon, G. H.: "Ocular Measurements," *Trans. Am. Med. Ass.*, 1928.

5 Ames, A., Jr., Ogle, K. N.., and Gliddon, G. H.: "Corresponding Retinal Points, the Horopter and Size and Shape of Ocular Images," *J. Opt. Soc. Am.*, Oct., Nov., 1932.

6 Anderson, J. Ringland: "Ocular Vertical Deviations."

7 Atwood, W. H.: "Concise Comparative Anatomy."

*8 Balado, –, and Franke, –: *Das Corpus Geniculatum.* Berlin, 1937.

9 Bannister, H.: "Some Discussion on Vision," page 227.

10 Bannon, R. E.: *Columbia Opto.*, 1949.

11 Bárány, E. H.: and Halldén, U.: *Acta. Physiol. Scand.*, Vol. XIV.

12 Bárány, E. H., and Halldén, U.: *Abst. Ophth. Lit.*, I, 1569.

13 Bartlett, F. C.: "Report on a Joint Discussion on Vision by the Physical and Optical Societies, 1932," page 237.

14 Bender, M. B., and Savitsky, N.: *Arch. Ophth.*, XXIII, 1046.

15 Bender, M. B., and Weinstein, E. A.: *Arch. Neurol. and Psych.*, XLIX, 98.

16 Bielchowsky, A.: *Am. J. Ophth.*, XXI, 843.

17 Bielchowsky, A.: "Dissociated Divergence," *Arch. f. Ophth.*, CXXV, 493.

18 Bielchowsky, A.: "Lectures on Motor Anomalies of the Eyes," *Arch. Ophth.*, XII, 802.

19 Blumenfeld, W.: "Untersuchungen über die Scheinbare Grösse in Sehraum," *Z. f. Psychol. u. Physiol. der Sinnesorgane*, LXV, 241.

20 Boeder, P.: personal communication.

*21 Brouwer, B.: *Zeitschr f. d. ges. Neurol. u. Psychiat.*, XL, 152.

22 Bruce, G. M.: *Arch. Ophth.*, XIII, 639.

23 Burian, H.: "The Rôle of Peripheral Fusion in Orthoptic Training," *Am. J. Ophth.*, XXX, 1005.

24 Buzzard, E., Farquhar: *Proc. Roy. Soc. Med., Neuro. Section*, I, 83.

25 Cantonnet, A., and Filliozat, J.: "Strabismus,"

26 Charnwood, Lord: *Brit. Orth. J.*, 1950.

27 Charnwood, Lord:. "Notes on Prolonged Occlusion," *Optician*, Aug. 8th, 1947.

28 Charnwood, Lord: "Observations on Ocular Dominance," *Optician*, Aug. 19th, 1949.

29 Charnwood, Lord: "Some Factors affecting Physiological Diplopia," *Optician*, Jan. 6th, 1950.

30 Charnwood, Lord: *Trans. Lond. Ref. Hosp. Jubilee Cong.*, 1947.

31 Charnwood, Lord: "Panum's Fusional Areas," *Optician*, May 19th, 1950.

32 Charnwood, Lord: "Diagnostic and Theurapeutic Use of Monocular Occlusion," B.O.A. Lond. Opt. Cong., 1950.

33 Charnwood, Lord: *Nature*, Vol. CLXVI, 348.

34 Charnwood, Lord: in preparation.

35 Charnwood, Lord: *Proc. S.M.C. Con.*, 1948.

36 Chavasse, F. B.: "Worth's Squint," 7th ed., 1939.

37 Cheshire, R. W.: personal communication.
Clark: see Le Gros Clark.

38 Cogan, D. G.: "Neurology of Ocular Muscles," Pub. Charles C. Thompson.

39 Colenbrander, M. C.: *Ned. Tidj. Genees.*, I, 809.

40 Colson, Z.: *J. Am. Med. Ass.*, CXV, 1525.

41 Cooper, Sybil, and Daniel, P. M.: *Brain*, LXXII, I, 1.

42 Cooper, Sybil, Daniel, P. M., and Whitteridge, D.: *J. Physiol.*, CVIII, 41.

42*a* Cooper, Sybil, Daniel, P. M., and Whitteridge, D.: *J. Physiol.*, CIX.

43 Corbin, K. B., and Harrison, F.: *J. Comp. Neurol.*, LXXVII, 187.

44 Corbin, K. B., and Oliver, R. K.: *J. Comp. Neurol.*, LXXVII, 171.

*45 Cuajunco, F.: Contr. Embryol., Carnegie Inst.; CLXXIII, 97.

46 Danis, P. C.: *Am. J. Ophth.*, XXXI, 122.

47 Davson, H.: "Physiology of the Eye," Pub. Churchill, 1949.

48 Duke-Elder, Sir: *Lancet*, CCXVIII, 824.

49 Duke-Elder, Sir: "Textbook of Ophthalmology," Vol. I, 295ff, 1059.

50 Duke-Elder, Sir: "Textbook of Ophthalmology," Vol. 4, 3875.

50*a* Duke-Elder, Sir: "Textbook of Ophthalmology," Vol. 4, 3856.

51 Dunphy, E. B.: *Am. J. Ophth.*, XI, 298.

52 Dusser de Barenne, J. G., and McCulloch, W. S.: *J. Neurophysiol.*, I, 69.

53 Ellerbrook, V. J.: *Am. J. Optom.*, XXVI, 530.

54 Elliman, H.: *Optician*, Dec. 24th, 1948.
Elliman, H.: *Optician*, Feb. 11th, 1949.

55 Elliman, H.: *Refractionist*, May, 1939.

56 Evans, C. S. Lovatt; personal communication.

57 Fincham, E. F.: *B. J. Ophth.*, *Monograph Supplement No. VIII.*

58 Fincham, E. F.: personal communication.

59 Ford, F. R., and Walsh, F. B.: *Arch. Ophth.*, XXIII, 1274.

60 Forster, L.: *J. Physiol.*, XXVIII, 201.

60*a* Forster, L.: *Arch. Ophth.*, XXXIII, 362.

61 Francis, J. L., and Harwood, K. A.: Research in progress.

62 Frank, C.: *J. f. Psychol. u. Neurol.*, XXVI, 200.

64 Giles, G. H.: "The Practice of Orthoptics." 1943.

65 Glees, P.: *J. Anat.*, LXXV, 434.

65*a* Glees, P.: *J. Anat.*, LXXVI, 313.

65*b* Grahe, K.: *Acta Oto-Lary*, XXVI, 268.

66 Granit, R.: "The Sensory Mechanism of the Retina," Pub. Oxford University Press.

67 Hartridge, H.: "The Perception of Fine Detail," *Trans. Roy. Soc.*, No. 592.

68 Hartridge, H.: "Recent Advances in the Physiology of Vision," Pub. Churchill.

69 Hartridge, H., and Thomson, L. C.: *Brit. J. Ophth.*, XXXII, 581.
70 Helmholtz, H. von: "Treatise on Physiological Optics," Translated by J. Southall, Opt. Soc. Am., 1925.
71 Hines, M.: *Am. J. Anat.*, XLVII, 1.
72 Hirsch, M. J., and Weymouth, F. L.: *Arch. Ophth.*, XXXIX, 210.
73 Hoessly, G. F.: *Abst. Ophth. Lit.*, I, 2259.
74 Holmes, G. B.: *B. J. Ophth.*, V, 241.
75 Holmes, G. B.: *B.M.J.*, July 16th, 1938.
75*a* Ittelson, W. H., and Ames, A., Jr.: *J. Psychol.*, XXX, 43.
76 Jefferson, G.: *B.M.J.*, June 25th, 1949.
76*a* Kompanejetz, S.: *Acta Oto-Laryn.*, XII, 332.
77 Kleyn, A. de, and Versteegh, C.: *J. Laryn. and Otol.*, XLII, 649.
78 Kulchitsky, N.: *J. Anat.*, XLIX, 1.
*79 Kundt, A.: *Poggendorffs Annalen*, CXX.
80 Lancaster, W. B., "Fifty Years' Experience of Ocular Motility," *Am. J. Ophth.*, XXIV.
81 Langlands, –: *Trans. Opt. Soc.*, XXVII, 45, 83.
83 Le Gros Clark, W. E.: *Brit. J. Ophth.*, XVI, 264.
84 Le Gros Clark, W. E.: *Brit. J. Ophth.*, LVI, 264.
85 Le Gros Clark, W. E.: *J. Anat.*, LXXV, 225.
86 Le Gros Clark, W. E.: *J. Anat.*, LXXVI, 369.
87 Le Gros Clark, W. E.: *Trans. Oxford Ophth. Con.*, 1942.
88 Le Gros Clark, W. E., and Glees, P.: *J. Anat.*, LXXV, 295.
89 Le Gros Clark, W. E., and Northfield, D. W.: *Brain*, LX, 126.
90 Le Gros Clark, W. E., and Penman, G. G.: *Proc. Roy. Soc.*, B, CXIV, 291.
91 Le Gros Clark, W. E., and Sunderland, S.: *J. Anat.*, LXXIII, 563.
92 Le Gros Clark, W. E., and Sunderland, S.: *Proc. Roy. Soc.*, B, CXIV, 291.
93 Lockhart, R. D., and Brandt, W.: *J. Anat.*, LXXII, 470.
94 Lord, M. A., and Wright, W. D.: *Nature*, CLXII, 25.
94*a* Lord, M. A., and Wright, W. D.: *Nature*, CLXIII, 803.
*95 Lotze, H.: "Medische Psychologie," Leipzig, 1852.
96 Luneburg, R. K.: "A Mathematical Analysis of Binocular Vision," Princeton University Press for the Dartmouth Eye Institute, 1947.
97 Lyle, T. K., and Jackson, S.: "Practical Orthoptics in the Treatment of Squint," 3rd. ed., Pub. H. K. Lewis, 1949.
98 Marlow, F. W.: *Arch. Ophth.*, XIX, 194.
99 Marlow, F. W.: "The Relative Position of Rest of the Eyes and the Prolonged Occlusion Test," Philadelphia, 1924.
100 Matteuci, P.: *Ophthalmologica*, CXIV, 377.
101 McColl, L.: "Servomechanisms," Pub. Van Nostrand, 1945.
102 Mein, J.: *Brit. J. Orth.*, 1950.
103 Minchowski, M.: Schw. *Arch. f. Neu. u. Psych.*, VI, 201.
104 Moreu, P.: *Abst. Ophth. Lit.*, II, 567.
105 Mott, F. W., and Schäffer, E. A.: *Brain*, XIII, 165.
106 Murroughs, T. R., and Christakos, J.: *Optician*, Nov. 18th, 1949.
107 Nicholson, H.: *J. Comp. Neuro.*, XXXVII, 31.
108 Ogle, K. N.: "An Analytical Treatment of the Longitudinal Horopter," *J. Opt. Soc. Am.*, XXII, 665.

109 Ogle, K. N.: "The Induced Size Effect," *Arch. Ophth.*, XX, 604.

110 Panum, P. L.: Physiologische untersuchungen über das Sehen mit zwei Augen.

112 Powell, W. H.: *J. Aviation Med.*, IX, 97.

113 Polyak, S.: "The Retina".

113*a* Polyak, S.: *Univ. Calif. Pub. Anat.*, II, 1.

114 Quick, R. J: *Optician*, Sept. 30th, 1949.

115 Rademaker, G. G. J., and Ter Braak, J. W. G.: *Brain*, LXXI, 48.

116 Reese, W. S., and Yaskin, J. C.: *Am. J. Ophth.*, XXIV, 544.

117 Rochon-Duvigneand, A.: "Les Yeux et la Vision des Vertebres."

118 Roper, K., and Bannon, R. E.: *Arch. Ophth.*, XXXI, 338.

120 Russel, R.: *J. Physiol.*, XVII, 1.

121 Schäffer, E. A.: *Brain*, XI, 1.

122 Schäffer, H., and Erner, F.: *F.I.A.T.* No. 1176.

123 Sedan, J., and Sedan-Bauby, S.: "Physiopathology of Artificially Induced Diplopias," *Arch. d'Ophth.*, VIII, 233.

124 Sedan, J., and Sedan-Bauby, S.: *Abst. Ophth. Lit.*, II, 1261.

125 Sherrington, C. S.: "The Integrative Action of the Nervous System."

126 Sherrington, C. S.: *J. Physiol.*, XVII, 211.

127 Spiegel, E. A.: *Arch. Neurol. and Psychiat.*, XXIX, 1084.

128 Spiegel, E. A., and Scala, N. P.: *Arch. Ophth.*, XVIII, 614.

129 *Strand Magazine*, Feb., 1950.

130 Tozer, F. M., and Sherrington, C. S.: *Proc. Roy. Soc.*, LXXXII, 450.

131 Tschermak, A., von Seysenegg: Handbuch der Physiol., Vol. XII, II, pp. 854ff.

131*a* Tschermak, A., von Seysenegg: Handbuch der Physiol., Vol. XII, II, pp. 988ff.

*132 Turing, –.: *J. Lond. Math. Soc.*, II, 42, 230.

134 Van der Velden, H. A.: *Ophthalmologica*, CXI, 321.

135 Verhoeff, F.: *Arch. Ophth*, X, 640, I.

136 Verhoeff, F.: "New Theory of Stereoscopic Vision" *Arch. Ophth.*, XIII, 151.

137 Verhoeff, F.: *Arch. Ophth.*, XXV, 780.

138 Verhoeff, F.: *Ophth. Rec.*, X, 300.

*139 Volkmann, A. W.: Das Sehen, 1846.

*140 Volkmann, A. W.: Physiologische untersuchungen im Gebiete der Optik, Chap. I; Leipzig, 1864.

141 Walls, G.: *Arch. Ophth.*, XVIII, 912.

142 Walshe, F. M.: *Brain*, XLIV, 539.

142*a* Warman, Royce, J.: *Optician*, Sept. 23rd, 1949.

143 Watchurst, G. R.: awaiting publication.

144 Watchurst, G. R.: personal communication.

145 Wiener, N.: "Cybernetics," Pub. Wiley and Sons, Inc., 1948.

*146 Wiener, N., and Rosenblueth, A.: "Conduction of the Impulses in Cardiac Muscles," *Arch. Inst. Cardiol.* Mexico, XVI, 205.

147 Wilkison, H. J.: *Med. J. Australia*, 1929, II, 768.

148 Winkelman, J. E.: *B. J. Ophth.*, XXXIII, 629.

149 Winkelman, J. E.: *Ophthalmologica*, CXV, 62.

150 Wolff, E.: "Anatomy of the Eye and Orbit," Pub. H. K. Lewis.

151 Woodworth, R. S.: "Psychology. A Study of Mental Life." Pub. Menthuen. 12th ed.

152 Woolard, H. H.: *J. Anat.*, LXV, 215.

153 Woolard, H. H.: *Trans. O.S.U.K.*, LVII, 84.

154 Worth, C.: "Squint. Its Causes, Pathology and Treatment."

155 Wright, W. D.: awaiting publication.

156 Wright, W. D.: personal communication.

157 Wright, W. D.: *Proc. S.M.C. Con.*, 1948.

158 Wright, W. D.: "Researches on Normal and Defective Colour Vision." Pub. Henry Kimpton, 1946.

*159 Wundt, W.: Theorie des Sinneswahrnehmung, 1862.

INDEX

DATE DUE

JAN 8 1973				
DEC 7 1972				
MAR 21 1975				
MAR 9 1975				
JAN 6 1986				
NOV 28 1988				
NOV 28 1988				